DIABETES
Friendly Kitchen

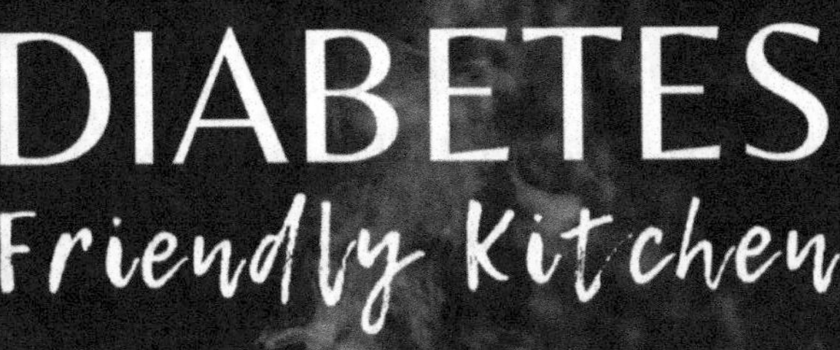

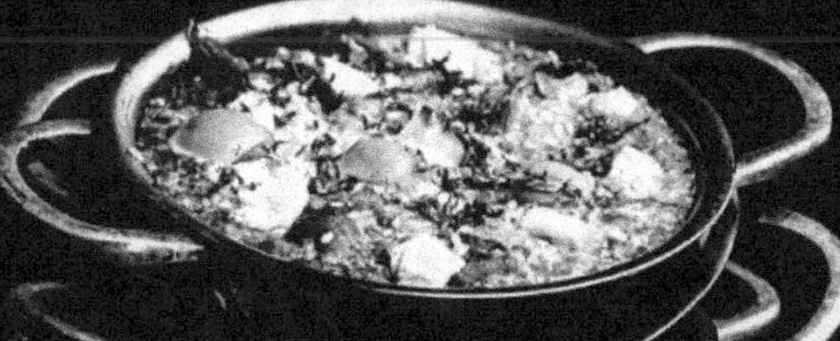

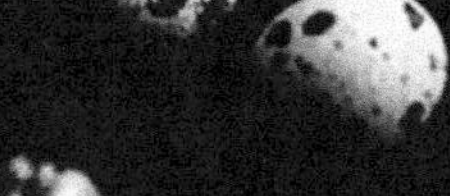

Dave Kesh

Table of Contents

Introduction

Understanding Diabetes

Diabetes is a chronic disorder that affects the way the body controls blood sugar, commonly known as glucose. It happens when the body either does not create enough insulin or cannot adequately utilize the insulin it produces. Insulin is a hormone that helps transfer glucose from the circulation into cells to be utilized for energy.

There are various forms of diabetes, including type 1, type 2, and gestational diabetes. Type 1 diabetes is an autoimmune illness in which the immune system erroneously assaults and kills the insulin-producing cells in the pancreas. People with type 1 diabetes need daily insulin injections or the use of an insulin pump to regulate their blood sugar levels.

Type 2 diabetes is the most prevalent type of diabetes and is commonly related with lifestyle factors such as obesity and physical inactivity. In type 2 diabetes, the body develops resistant to the effects of insulin, resulting to high blood sugar levels. This form of diabetes may typically be treated with lifestyle changes such as adopting a nutritious diet, increasing physical exercise, and decreasing weight if required. In certain circumstances, medication or insulin treatment may also be necessary.

Gestational diabetes arises during pregnancy and affects roughly 2-10% of pregnant women. It normally disappears after delivery, but women who have had gestational diabetes have an increased chance of getting type 2 diabetes later in life.

Managing diabetes with a nutritious diet is vital for maintaining stable blood sugar levels and minimizing complications. A healthy diabetic diet focuses on balancing carbs, proteins, and lipids while also consuming lots of fruits, vegetables, and whole grains. Carbs have the most significant influence on blood sugar levels, thus it is crucial to pick carbs that are rich in fiber and have a lower glycemic index.

Meal planning plays a critical part in controlling diabetes efficiently. It helps patients with diabetes establish realistic objectives and build a balanced diet plan that fits their nutritional requirements while keeping blood sugar levels in line. Meal planning also helps people make better food choices, limit portion sizes, and keep a regular eating pattern.

In addition to carbs, proteins and lipids also have a role in blood sugar regulation. Proteins help slow down the absorption of carbs, limiting fast rises in blood sugar levels. Choosing lean sources of protein such as chicken, fish, tofu, and lentils is suggested.

Healthy fats, such as those found in avocados, almonds, and olive oil, are especially helpful for those with diabetes. They increase insulin sensitivity and boost heart health. However, portion management is vital while taking fats since they are calorie-dense.

Fiber is another crucial component for diabetes individuals. It helps manage blood sugar levels, enhance digestion, and increase fullness. High-fiber foods include vegetables, whole grains, fruits, and legumes.

When preparing meals for diabetes patients, it is vital to employ healthy cooking techniques such as grilling, roasting, steaming, and sautéing. These approaches help keep the nutrients in the meal without adding extra fats or sweets. Reducing additional sugars in recipes is also crucial, and natural sweeteners may be used as alternatives.

This knowledge of diabetes and the necessity of a balanced diet sets the basis for efficient meal planning and cooking skills that cater to the unique nutritional demands of those with diabetes. By following a well-balanced meal plan and making sensible food choices, persons with diabetes may successfully regulate their blood sugar levels and enjoy a healthy lifestyle.

Types of Diabetes

Diabetes is a chronic disorder that impairs the body's capacity to control blood sugar, or glucose. There are various forms of diabetes, each with its own origins, symptoms, and treatment techniques.

1. Type 1 Diabetes: Type 1 diabetes is an autoimmune illness in which the immune system erroneously assaults and kills the insulin-producing cells in the pancreas. This leads in a lack of insulin synthesis, resulting to high blood sugar levels. Type 1 diabetes generally develops in infancy or adolescence, however it may occur at any age. People with type 1 diabetes need daily insulin injections or the use of an insulin pump to regulate their blood sugar levels.

2. Type 2 Diabetes: Type 2 diabetes is the most prevalent type of diabetes and is commonly related

with lifestyle factors such as obesity and physical inactivity. In type 2 diabetes, the body develops resistance to the effects of insulin, resulting in high blood sugar levels. Initially, the pancreas may create additional insulin to compensate for this resistance, but with time, insulin production may diminish. Type 2 diabetes may frequently be treated with lifestyle changes such as adopting a nutritious diet, increasing physical exercise, and decreasing weight if required. In certain circumstances, medication or insulin treatment may also be necessary.

3. Gestational Diabetes: Gestational diabetes arises during pregnancy and affects a tiny number of pregnant women. It is caused by hormonal changes that impair insulin sensitivity. Gestational diabetes normally resolves after delivery, but women who have had gestational diabetes have an increased chance of having type 2 diabetes later in life. Blood sugar levels during pregnancy should be managed for the health of both the mother and the baby.

It is crucial to emphasize that whereas type 1 and type 2 diabetes are chronic illnesses that need continuing treatment, gestational diabetes is transient and normally disappears after delivery.

Each form of diabetes needs distinct care measures to maintain stable blood sugar levels and avoid complications. This frequently needs a mix of medicine, insulin therapy, lifestyle adjustments, and regular monitoring of blood sugar levels.

Understanding the various forms of diabetes is vital for persons with diabetes and their healthcare professionals to design an effective treatment strategy. By properly controlling blood sugar levels with medication, lifestyle adjustments, and a nutritious diet, persons with diabetes may have a happy and healthy life.

Managing Diabetes with a Healthy Diet

One of the major components in controlling diabetes, regardless of the type, is keeping a balanced diet. A nutritious diet may help patients with diabetes maintain their blood sugar levels, manage their weight, and lower the risk of complications associated with the illness.

When it comes to controlling diabetes with a healthy diet, there are numerous crucial variables to consider:

1. Carbohydrate Counting: Carbohydrates have the most significant influence on blood sugar levels. It is vital for patients with diabetes to control their carbohydrate consumption and spread it properly throughout the day. This may be done by carbohydrate counting, which entails measuring the quantity of carbs in each meal and modifying insulin or medicine dosages appropriately.

2. Choosing the Right carbs: Not all carbs are made equal. Complex carbs, such as whole grains, legumes, and vegetables, are absorbed more slowly and have a milder influence on blood sugar levels compared to simple carbohydrates like sugary snacks and beverages. It is advisable to concentrate on ingesting complex carbs while minimizing or avoiding simple carbohydrates.

3. Portion Control: Controlling portion sizes is vital for regulating blood sugar levels and keeping a healthy weight. Overeating may lead to surges in blood sugar levels, while habitually eating too little may result in low blood sugar levels. It is vital to talk with a healthcare physician or a qualified dietitian to establish proper portion amounts for meals and snacks.

4. Balancing Macronutrients: In addition to carbs, it is vital to have enough quantities of protein and healthy fats in the diet. Protein helps with satiety and may help normalize blood sugar levels. Healthy fats, such as those found in avocados, almonds, and olive oil, may help improve insulin sensitivity and decrease inflammation.

5. Fiber-Rich Foods: Including fiber-rich foods in the diet is advantageous for those with diabetes. Fiber slows down the digestion and absorption of carbs, resulting in more stable blood sugar levels. It also helps with weight control, maintains digestive health, and decreases the risk of heart disease. Best sources of fiber include fruits, vegetables, whole grains, legumes, and nuts.

6. Regular Meal Timing: Establishing regular meal timings and spacing meals evenly throughout the day will help manage blood sugar levels. It is vital to avoid skipping meals or spending lengthy periods without eating, since this might lead to abnormalities in blood sugar levels.

7. Limiting Added Sugars: Consuming excessive quantities of added sugars may lead to rises in blood sugar levels and contribute to weight gain. It is vital to read food labels and be careful of hidden

sugars in processed foods and drinks. Opting for natural sweeteners like stevia or using modest quantities of honey or maple syrup might be healthier options.

It is crucial for patients with diabetes to engage closely with their healthcare physician or a certified dietitian to design a tailored meal plan that takes into consideration their unique dietary requirements, tastes, and lifestyle. Regular monitoring of blood sugar levels and modifications to the diet may be essential to maintain stable blood sugar management.

Managing diabetes with a nutritious diet is vital for persons afflicted with the illness. A nutritious diet consisting of whole foods, fruits, vegetables, lean meats, and healthy fats may help manage blood sugar levels, lower the risk of problems associated with diabetes, and improve overall health. It is crucial to engage with a registered dietitian or healthcare practitioner to design a tailored meal plan that suits your particular requirements and interests. Additionally, combining regular physical exercise and monitoring blood sugar levels may further boost the efficiency of a balanced diet in treating diabetes. By making lifestyle adjustments and adopting a balanced diet, persons with diabetes may live a better and happier life.

Meal Planning for Diabetic Patients

Importance of Meal Planning

Meal planning is of essential significance for a diabetic patient as it plays a critical part in maintaining blood sugar levels, boosting general health, and reducing problems connected with diabetes. Here are some important reasons why meal planning is vital for those with diabetes:

1. Blood Sugar Control: Consistently monitoring and regulating blood sugar levels is the main objective for those with diabetes. Meal planning provides for greater control over carbohydrate consumption, which has the most significant influence on blood sugar levels. By preparing meals in advance, people may guarantee that they are getting the proper quantity of carbs, proteins, and fats, and distribute them equally throughout the day. This helps minimize spikes or decreases in blood sugar levels, increasing stability and minimizing the risk of hyperglycemia or hypoglycemia.

2. Weight Management: Maintaining a healthy weight is vital for controlling diabetes efficiently.

Meal planning enables consumers to regulate portion sizes and make better food choices, which may benefit in weight management. By integrating a balanced diet with optimal calorie consumption, people may reach and maintain a healthy weight, minimizing the risk of obesity-related problems such as heart disease and insulin resistance.

3. Nutritional Balance: Diabetes demands careful attention to nutritional intake, since specific nutrients play a critical role in regulating the illness. Meal planning assists people to ensure they are obtaining enough levels of key nutrients such vitamins, minerals, fiber, and antioxidants. By include a range of nutrient-dense foods in their meal plans, people may promote their overall health and well-being.

4. Personalized Approach: Each person with diabetes has distinct nutritional demands, preferences, and lifestyle circumstances that need to be taken into consideration. Meal planning provides for a tailored approach to treating diabetes, ensuring that the individual's unique needs are satisfied. Working with a healthcare physician or registered dietitian may assist build a meal plan suited to an individual's personal

requirements, making it simpler to stick to the plan and achieve optimum outcomes.

5. tension Reduction: Diabetes treatment may be daunting, and meal planning can help ease some of the tension involved with making daily dietary decisions. Having a well-thought-out meal plan in place avoids the need to continually think about what to eat, decreases choice fatigue, and offers a feeling of order and control. This may help to greater adherence to dietary restrictions and overall diabetes control.

Meal planning is an important component of treating diabetes efficiently. It assists people to maintain stable blood sugar levels, regulate their weight, assure sufficient nutrition, and minimize stress associated with food choices. By designing a tailored meal plan in cooperation with healthcare specialists, persons with diabetes may take control of their condition and enhance their overall health and well-being.

Dangers of not Planning meals

Not preparing meals for diabetes individuals might have serious hazards and repercussions. Here are some important reasons why not preparing meals might be bad for those with diabetes:

1. Blood Sugar Instability: Without a meal plan, diabetes patients may eat uneven quantities of carbs, proteins, and fats, leading to unexpected variations in blood sugar levels. This might result in frequent spikes or decreases in blood sugar, raising the risk of hyperglycemia or hypoglycemia. Uncontrolled blood sugar levels may have major health repercussions and lead to long-term difficulties such as nerve damage, renal disease, and cardiovascular problems.

2. Poor Nutritional Intake: Without an organized meal plan, diabetes patients may struggle to eat a balanced diet that satisfies their nutritional demands. This may lead to shortages in critical nutrients such vitamins, minerals, fiber, and antioxidants. Inadequate nutrition may weaken the immune system, hinder wound healing, and raise the risk of infections and other issues linked with diabetes.

3. Weight Management Challenges: Without meal planning, it may be difficult for diabetes patients to regulate portion sizes and make appropriate food choices regularly. This might lead to weight gain or difficulties in maintaining a healthy weight. Obesity is a major risk factor for diabetes and may

aggravate insulin resistance, making blood sugar management even more problematic.

4. Increased tension and worry: Not having a meal plan in place may induce tension and worry for diabetes individuals. The frequent need to make on-the-spot judgments regarding what to eat may be burdensome and contribute to decision fatigue. This stress may significantly effect mental well-being and possibly disrupt adherence to food rules and overall diabetes control.

5. Lack of Accountability and Monitoring: Without a defined meal plan, it becomes tough to monitor and track food consumption effectively. This might make it difficult to recognize trends or events that may alter blood sugar levels. Additionally, without accountability, it is easier for diabetes patients to depart from their suggested dietary limits, leading to uncontrolled blood sugar levels and greater risk of complications.

Not arranging meals for diabetes individuals might have significant hazards and repercussions. It might result in unstable blood sugar levels, poor dietary intake, weight control issues, increased stress, and lack of responsibility and monitoring. It is vital for persons with diabetes to prioritize meal planning and engage with healthcare experts to build a tailored meal plan that meets their unique requirements and promotes optimum diabetes control.

Setting Realistic Goals

Setting realistic objectives for a diabetic patient's meal plan is vital for their general health and well-being. Here are some crucial elements to consider while developing feasible goals:

1. Individualized Approach: Each diabetes patient is unique, with various food choices, lifestyle circumstances, and medical concerns. It is vital to take these aspects into consideration when establishing objectives for their diet plan. By adapting the objectives to their unique requirements and circumstances, it raises the probability of success and adherence.

2. Gradual adjustments: Making abrupt adjustments to a diabetic patient's food plan may be burdensome and unsustainable. Instead, it is crucial to concentrate on modest adjustments that may be adopted over time. This technique helps the patient to acclimate to new eating habits and enhances the probability of long-term success.

3. Realistic Expectations: Setting attainable objectives is vital for keeping motivation and reducing discouragement. It is crucial to create reasonable expectations that are feasible for the patient. This may entail breaking down big objectives into smaller, more doable tasks. Celebrating little triumphs along the road may help improve motivation and promote continuing growth.

4. knowledge and assistance: Providing diabetes patients with the proper knowledge and assistance is crucial for goal attainment. This might involve educating kids about portion management, carbohydrate counting, label reading, and making better food choices. Additionally, delivering continuous support via frequent check-ins, counseling sessions, or group education programs may help patients remain on track and handle any issues they may experience.

5. Flexibility and Adaptability: Diabetes treatment is a lifetime endeavor, and objectives may need to be changed over time. It is crucial to stress flexibility and adaptation in the meal plan to meet changes in the patient's health, lifestyle, or personal circumstances. This allows for continual

improvement and ensures that the objectives stay relevant and feasible.

6. Monitoring and assessment: Regular monitoring and assessment of the meal plan's efficacy is vital for success. This may entail measuring blood sugar levels, weight, and other important health indicators. By routinely monitoring progress, healthcare professionals may make necessary modifications to the meal plan and ensure that the objectives stay reasonable and attainable.

Creating a Balanced Meal Plan

Creating a balanced diet plan for a diabetic patient is vital for maintaining their blood sugar levels and general health. Here are some crucial elements to consider when designing a balanced meal plan:

1. Carbohydrate Counting: Carbohydrates have the most significant influence on blood sugar levels, thus it is vital to include them in the meal plan in regulated quantities. Carbohydrate counting entails tracking the quantity of carbs ingested and distributing them equally throughout the day. This helps to reduce spikes and dips in blood sugar levels.

2. Portion Control: Controlling portion sizes is vital for regulating calorie intake and keeping a healthy weight. It is necessary to educate the diabetes patient on optimal portion sizes for various dietary categories, such as grains, proteins, fruits, vegetables, and fats. This helps them get a balanced and nutrient-dense supper.

3. contain a range of Nutrient-Dense meals: A balanced meal plan should contain a range of nutrient-dense meals to supply necessary vitamins, minerals, and fiber. This involves eating whole grains, lean meats, fruits, veggies, and healthy fats throughout each meal. These foods assist to increase satiety, normalize blood sugar levels, and improve general health.

4. restrict Added Sugars and Processed meals: Diabetic patients should restrict their intake of added sugars and processed meals, since they may contribute to fast rises in blood sugar levels. Instead, concentrate on complete, unprocessed meals that are low in added sugars and abundant in nutrients. This includes picking fresh fruits over sweet treats and opting for nutritious grains instead of processed carbs.

5. Balance Macronutrients: A balanced meal plan should contain a balance of macronutrients - carbs, proteins, and fats. Each macronutrient serves a critical function in maintaining stable blood sugar levels and supporting overall health. It is crucial to educate the patient on the necessity of incorporating all three macronutrients in their meals and snacks.

6. Regular Meal Times and Consistency: Establishing regular meal times and keeping consistency in the meal plan is helpful for regulating blood sugar levels. Diabetic patients should attempt to consume meals and snacks at predictable intervals throughout the day to help maintain their blood sugar levels. This also helps to avoid overeating or missing meals, which may lead to abnormalities in blood sugar levels.

7. Fluid Intake: Adequate hydration is vital for general health, including blood sugar regulation. Encourage the diabetic patient to drink lots of water throughout the day and restrict sugary drinks. Water helps to maintain optimum hydration, promotes digestion, and may help reduce hunger.

By following these suggestions it will enhance your overall health and well-being.

Essential Nutrients for Diabetic Patients

Carbohydrates and Blood Sugar Control

Carbohydrates are an important ingredient found in numerous diets, including grains, fruits, vegetables, and dairy products. When taken, carbohydrates are broken down into glucose, which is the major source of energy for the body. However, for persons with diabetes, regulating carbohydrate consumption is critical for blood sugar management.

Carbohydrates have the most substantial influence on blood sugar levels compared to proteins and lipids. This is because they are immediately turned into glucose and absorbed into the circulation. Therefore, persons with diabetes need to watch their carbohydrate consumption and distribute it evenly throughout the day to minimize spikes and dips in blood sugar levels.

One approach often used for carbohydrate monitoring is carbohydrate counting. This entails assessing the quantity of carbs taken in a meal or snack and modifying insulin dosages appropriately. By carefully managing carbohydrate consumption, persons with diabetes may better regulate their blood sugar levels and avoid hyperglycemia (high blood sugar) or hypoglycemia (low blood sugar).

It is crucial to recognize that not all carbs are created equal. There are two basic kinds of carbs: simple carbohydrates and complicated carbohydrates. Simple carbohydrates, commonly known as sugars, are present in meals such as candy, soda, and baked goods. They are easily absorbed and may produce abrupt rises in blood sugar levels. On the other hand, complex carbs, found in whole grains, legumes, and vegetables, are absorbed more slowly, resulting in a steady rise in blood sugar levels.

When creating a balanced diet for a diabetic patient, it is vital to concentrate on adding complex carbs rather than simple carbohydrates. Whole grains, such as brown rice, quinoa, and whole wheat bread, give more fiber and minerals compared to refined grains. Fiber helps slow down the digestion of carbs and may help manage blood sugar levels.

In addition to carbohydrate restriction, it is crucial to consider meal sizes while maintaining blood sugar levels. Controlling portion sizes helps to regulate calorie intake and maintain a healthy weight. Educating the diabetic patient on optimal portion sizes for various food categories is vital for creating a balanced meal.

Furthermore, it is vital to highlight that blood sugar regulation is not simply reliant on carbs. Protein and fat consumption also have a role in blood sugar regulation. Including lean proteins, such as chicken, fish, tofu, and lentils, in meals may help regulate blood sugar levels and enhance fullness. Healthy fats, such as avocados, almonds, and olive oil, may also help slow down the digestion of carbs and reduce blood sugar increases.

Recognizing the link between carbs and blood sugar regulation is critical for patients with diabetes. By monitoring carbohydrate consumption, concentrating on complex carbs, managing portion sizes, and integrating proteins and healthy fats, persons with diabetes may better regulate their blood sugar levels and enhance their overall health. Consulting with a healthcare expert or registered dietitian is suggested to establish a tailored meal plan that suits the particular requirements of each individual.

Types of Carbohydrates and their Impact on Blood Sugar Levels

Carbohydrates are a macronutrient present in diverse diets, and they have variable effects on blood sugar levels dependent on their makeup. There are two basic kinds of carbs: simple carbohydrates and complicated carbohydrates.

Simple carbohydrates, commonly known as sugars, are present in meals such as candy, soda, and baked goods. They are made up of one or two sugar molecules and are swiftly digested and absorbed into the circulation. As a consequence, they produce a fast spike in blood sugar levels. This may be troublesome for those with diabetes since it can lead to rises in blood sugar levels and possibly contribute to hyperglycemia.

On the other hand, complex carbohydrates are made up of three or more sugar molecules bonded together. They are present in foods such as whole grains, legumes, and vegetables. Complex carbs take longer to digest and are broken down into glucose more gradually, resulting in a slower rise in blood sugar levels. This delayed release of glucose helps to maintain stable blood sugar levels and is advantageous for those with diabetes.

Fiber is a significant component of complex carbohydrates. It is a form of carbohydrate that cannot be digested by the body. Fiber helps to slow down the digestion and absorption of carbs, which may help manage blood sugar levels. Foods rich in fiber, such as whole grains, fruits, vegetables, and legumes, are ideal options for those with diabetes since they give continuous energy and support stable blood sugar management.

It is vital for patients with diabetes to concentrate on including complex carbs into their diet rather than simple carbohydrates. Choosing whole grains over refined grains, such as brown rice instead of white rice or whole wheat bread instead of white bread, may deliver more fiber and minerals while limiting blood sugar rises.

When planning meals, it is also crucial to consider the glycemic index (GI) of carbohydrates. The glycemic index is a measure of how rapidly a carbohydrate-containing diet elevates blood sugar levels. Foods with a high GI, such as white bread and sugary snacks, induce a quick spike in blood sugar levels. On the other hand, meals with a low GI, such as whole grains and most vegetables, result in a slower and more gradual rise in blood sugar levels.

The kind of carbohydrates ingested may have a substantial influence on blood sugar levels. Simple carbohydrates, found in sweet meals, may produce quick rises in blood sugar levels, whereas complex carbs, found in whole grains, legumes, and vegetables, give sustained energy and encourage stable blood sugar management. Incorporating high-fiber meals and selecting carbs with a low glycemic index might further help blood sugar control for those with diabetes. Consulting with a healthcare expert or registered dietitian is suggested to establish a tailored meal plan that takes into account individual requirements and preferences.

Counting Carbohydrates

Counting carbs is a typical activity for patients with diabetes to regulate their blood sugar levels. It entails keeping track of the quantity of carbohydrates ingested in meals and snacks, since carbohydrates have the most significant influence on blood sugar levels compared to other macronutrients.

When counting carbs, persons with diabetes strive to eat a regular quantity of carbohydrates at each meal or snack to maintain stable blood sugar management. This allows individuals to better manage their prescription, such as insulin or oral medicines, and make necessary modifications depending on their carbohydrate consumption.

To count carbs efficiently, people need to understand the carbohydrate amount of different meals. Carbohydrate content may be detected on food labels, in carbohydrate counting books, or via internet tools. It is crucial to understand that carbs are not just contained in starchy meals like bread and rice but also in fruits, vegetables, dairy products, and even certain proteins like beans and lentils.

When calculating carbs, it is vital to consider portion proportions. varying foods have varying serving sizes and related carbohydrate quantities. For example, a piece of bread normally has approximately 15 grams of carbs, whereas a cup of cooked pasta may have around 45 grams. Measuring and measuring meal quantities may assist guarantee correct carbohydrate counts.

Once people establish the carbohydrate amount of their meals and snacks, they may utilize this knowledge to calculate their insulin or medicine dose as required. This is done in conjunction with a healthcare practitioner who may coach them on suitable insulin-to-carbohydrate ratios or medication modifications.

Counting carbs assists patients with diabetes to have better control over their blood sugar levels. By tracking their carbohydrate consumption, people may make educated dietary choices and modify their medicine appropriately. It helps patients prevent blood sugar spikes or drops, which may lead to issues and damage general health.

It is crucial to recognize that monitoring carbs is simply one part of diabetic treatment. Other variables such as physical activity, stress, and overall meal composition also have a role in blood sugar regulation. Therefore, persons with diabetes should engage with their healthcare team to build a complete diabetes management plan that includes carbohydrate tracking, regular physical exercise, medication management, and frequent blood sugar testing.

Measuring carbs is a beneficial technique for patients with diabetes to regulate their blood sugar levels successfully. By recognizing the carbohydrate amount of different foods and monitoring their consumption, people may make educated decisions and maintain stable blood sugar management. Consulting with healthcare specialists and having correct instruction on carbohydrate counting is vital for optimal diabetic control.

Glycemic Index and Glycemic Load

The glycemic index (GI) and glycemic load (GL) are two metrics that are used to analyze the influence of carbohydrates on blood sugar levels. They are often used by patients with diabetes to make educated meal choices and maintain their blood sugar control. The glycemic index is a grading system that provides a numerical value to carbohydrates based on how rapidly they elevate blood sugar levels relative to a reference meal, generally glucose or white bread. Carbohydrates having a high GI value are quickly digested and absorbed, generating a fast spike in blood sugar levels. On the other hand, carbohydrates with a low GI value are digested and absorbed more slowly, resulting in a slower and more gradual increase in blood sugar levels.

Foods having a high GI value include white bread, white rice, sugary snacks, and processed cereals. These foods may produce a significant surge in blood sugar levels and may lead to poor blood sugar management. Foods having a low GI rating include whole grains, fruits, vegetables, and legumes. These meals are processed more slowly, resulting in a more steady rise in blood sugar levels. The glycemic load takes into consideration both the glycemic index of a meal and the quantity of carbs in a serving. It gives a more precise indication of how a certain food or meal may affect blood sugar levels. The glycemic load is computed by multiplying the glycemic index of a food by the quantity of carbs in a serving and dividing it by 100.

For example, a watermelon has a high glycemic index but a low glycemic load since it contains a tiny quantity of carbs per serving. On the other hand, a baked potato has a high glycemic index and a high glycemic load since it includes a bigger quantity of carbs per serving. The glycemic index and glycemic load are measurements used to analyze the influence of carbohydrates on blood sugar levels. By knowing these metrics and making educated meal choices, persons with diabetes may better manage their blood sugar management.

Proteins and Diabetic Diet

Role of Proteins in Blood Sugar Management

Proteins have a key role in blood sugar regulation, particularly for those with diabetes. Unlike carbs, proteins have negligible influence on blood sugar levels since they do not directly elevate blood glucose levels. Instead, proteins are necessary for managing blood sugar levels and maintaining overall glycemic control.

When eaten, proteins are broken down into amino acids during digestion. These amino acids are subsequently utilized by the body to create and repair tissues, including muscles. This process consumes energy, which in turn helps to normalize blood sugar levels. Additionally, proteins have a satiating impact, meaning they assist to keep you feeling full for extended periods of time. This may be advantageous for those with diabetes who need to monitor their food intake and avoid blood sugar increases.

Furthermore, proteins have a lower glycemic index compared to carbs. This implies that they are digested and absorbed more slowly, resulting in a more steady release of glucose into the circulation. This helps to minimize rapid rises in blood sugar levels and supports improved glycemic control.

Including proper quantities of protein in meals and snacks may also assist to balance out the influence of carbs on blood sugar levels. When carbs are taken alone, they may induce a quick increase in blood glucose levels. However, when paired with protein, the digestion and absorption of carbs are slowed down, resulting to a more gradual release of glucose into the circulation.

It is vital to remember that the source and quality of protein are equally significant elements to consider. Lean forms of protein such as chicken, fish, tofu, lentils, and low-fat dairy products are often advised since they contain important nutrients without excessive quantities of saturated fats and cholesterol.

Proteins play a critical function in blood sugar regulation for persons with diabetes. They aid to manage blood sugar levels, increase satiety, and avoid rapid rises in blood glucose levels. By consuming proper quantities of protein in their diet, persons with diabetes may better manage their blood sugar management and overall glycemic health. However, it is crucial to maintain a balanced diet and collaborate with healthcare specialists to build a complete diabetes management plan that takes into consideration different aspects, including protein consumption.

Choosing Lean Sources of Protein

Choosing lean sources of protein is vital for maintaining a balanced diet and regulating blood sugar levels, particularly for persons with diabetes. Lean sources of protein are those that supply important nutrients without excessive quantities of saturated fats and cholesterol. Poultry, such as chicken and turkey, is a popular lean source of protein. These meats are lower in fat compared to red meats like beef and hog. Skinless chicken breast, in instance, is a lean alternative that is strong in protein and low in saturated fats.

Fish is another wonderful source for lean protein. Fatty fish like salmon, mackerel, and sardines are not only high in protein but also contain heart-healthy omega-3 fatty acids. These fatty acids have been demonstrated to offer several health advantages, including lowering inflammation and boosting heart health. Tofu is a plant-based protein source that is low in saturated fats and cholesterol. It is manufactured from soybeans and is a versatile ingredient that may be utilized in a number of cuisines. Tofu is also a good supply of key amino acids, making it a complete protein.

Legumes, such as beans, lentils, and chickpeas, are not only high in protein but also rich in fiber. They are a wonderful alternative for those with diabetes since they have a low glycemic index, meaning they have a little influence on blood sugar levels. Legumes may be added to soups, salads, or utilized as a meat alternative in numerous dishes. Low-fat dairy products like Greek yogurt, cottage cheese, and skim milk are also wonderful sources of lean protein. They give critical minerals such as calcium and vitamin D while being low in saturated fats. Greek yogurt, in example, is rich in protein and may be consumed on its own or used as a foundation for smoothies or sauces.

When picking lean sources of protein, it is crucial to consider the cooking techniques as well. Grilling, baking, steaming, or broiling meats are better alternatives compared to frying or breading them, which may add unneeded fats and calories. Selecting lean sources of protein is vital for those with diabetes to maintain a balanced diet and regulate blood sugar levels. Poultry, fish, tofu, lentils, and low-fat dairy products are all wonderful alternatives that supply necessary nutrients without excessive quantities of saturated fats and cholesterol. By integrating these lean proteins into their diets, persons with diabetes may enhance their overall glycemic management and promote better health.

Recommended Protein Intake for Diabetic Patients.

Protein is a vital macronutrient that plays a key role in sustaining overall health, particularly for those with diabetes. It aids in creating and repairing tissues, boosting immunological function, and controlling blood sugar levels. However, estimating the recommended protein consumption for diabetes patients may be problematic since it relies on different aspects such as age, sex, activity level, and general health.

The American Diabetes Association (ADA) says that patients with diabetes should strive for a moderate protein consumption, often about 15-20% of their total daily calorie intake. This advice coincides with the overall dietary requirements for the general population. However, it is crucial to remember that individual needs may differ, and it is preferable to contact a healthcare expert or qualified dietitian to assess the particular protein requirements. When evaluating protein sources for diabetes individuals, it is vital to pick lean ones that are low in saturated fats and cholesterol. As indicated previously, chicken, fish, tofu, lentils, and low-fat dairy products are wonderful alternatives. These sources supply high-quality protein while also delivering extra nutrients that assist overall wellness. It is also necessary to arrange protein consumption equally throughout the day to enhance blood sugar regulation. This may be done by consuming protein-rich meals in each meal and snack. For example, putting eggs or Greek yogurt into breakfast, adding chicken or fish to lunch and supper, and including lentils or tofu in vegetarian meals.

Recommended protein consumption for diabetes individuals should be modest and tailored depending on criteria such as age, sex, activity level, and general health. Choosing lean sources of protein, dividing protein consumption evenly throughout the day, and keeping a balanced diet are critical concerns for those with diabetes. By following these instructions, persons with diabetes may maintain their general health and efficiently control their blood sugar levels.

Healthy Fats and Diabetes

Understanding Different Types of Fats

Fats are an integral element of our diet and serve a critical function in sustaining overall health. However, not all fats are created equal, and it is crucial to understand the various kinds of fats and their consequences on our health.

1. Saturated fats: Saturated fats are normally solid at room temperature and are often found in animal products such as meat, butter, and full-fat dairy products. They may also be present in certain plant-based oils like coconut oil and palm oil. Consuming excessive quantities of saturated fats may elevate levels of LDL (low-density lipoprotein) cholesterol, which is generally referred to as "bad" cholesterol. High levels of LDL cholesterol may raise the risk of heart disease and stroke.

2. Trans fats: Trans fats are intentionally manufactured via a process called hydrogenation, which turns liquid vegetable oils into solid fats. Trans fats are typically found in processed meals, fried foods, baked products, and margarine. Like saturated fats, trans fats may raise LDL cholesterol levels and reduce HDL (high-density lipoprotein)

cholesterol levels, which is commonly referred to as "good" cholesterol. Therefore, it is advisable to restrict the intake of trans fats as much as possible.

3. Monounsaturated fats: Monounsaturated fats are considered heart-healthy lipids. They can help reduce LDL cholesterol levels and maintain or improve HDL cholesterol levels. Monounsaturated fats may be found in olive oil, avocados, nuts, and seeds. Including these items in your diet may have a good influence on heart health.

4. Polyunsaturated fats: Polyunsaturated fats are also considered heart-healthy fats. They may help decrease LDL cholesterol levels and offer necessary omega-3 and omega-6 fatty acids that our bodies cannot create on their own. Polyunsaturated fats may be found in fatty fish (such as salmon and trout), walnuts, flaxseeds, and soybean oil.

It is crucial to remember that although monounsaturated and polyunsaturated fats are typically regarded as better alternatives, moderation is still vital. Fats are abundant in calories, therefore taking them in excess may contribute to weight gain and other health complications. It is suggested to replace saturated and trans fats with better fats in your diet, rather than adding them on top of an existing high-fat diet.

When it comes to cooking and food preparation, it is also necessary to consider the smoke point of various kinds of fats. The smoke point is the temperature at which a lipid starts to break down and emit smoke. Using fats with a high smoke point, such as avocado oil or canola oil, for high-heat cooking techniques like frying or sautéing may help reduce the development of hazardous chemicals.

Recognizing the various kinds of fats and their consequences on our health is vital for making educated dietary decisions. Limiting the consumption of saturated and trans fats while introducing healthy choices like monounsaturated and polyunsaturated fats may assist boost heart health and general well-being. It is always suggested to speak with a healthcare expert or registered dietitian for tailored recommendations on fat consumption based on individual health requirements and objectives.

Incorporating Healthy Fats into the Diabetic Diet

Incorporating healthy fats into the diabetic diet is vital for maintaining general health and regulating blood sugar levels. While fats have been historically linked with detrimental health impacts, it is crucial to remember that not all fats are created equal. Healthy fats, such as monounsaturated and polyunsaturated fats, may offer several advantages for patients with diabetes.

Firstly, good fats may enhance heart health, which is particularly essential for persons with diabetes who are at a greater risk of developing cardiovascular issues. Monounsaturated fats, found in foods such as avocados, almonds, and olive oil, may help decrease harmful cholesterol levels and lessen the risk of heart disease.

Polyunsaturated fats, particularly omega-3 and omega-6 fatty acids, are also advantageous for patients with diabetes. These fats may help decrease inflammation in the body and promote brain function. Sources of omega-3 fatty acids include fatty fish like salmon and trout, whereas sources of omega-6 fatty acids include vegetable oils like soybean and sunflower oil.

Incorporating healthy fats into the diabetic diet might also benefit in blood sugar management. Fats slow down the digestion and absorption of carbs, resulting in a slower and more gradual increase in blood sugar levels after a meal. This may help reduce increases in blood sugar and encourage more consistent glucose levels throughout the day.

When introducing healthy fats into the diabetic diet, it is vital to concentrate on portion sizes and pick sources that are low in saturated and trans fats. Saturated fats, found in meals like red meat, full-fat dairy products, and tropical oils, may raise harmful cholesterol levels and should be reduced. Trans fats, frequently found in processed and fried meals, should be avoided completely since they have been linked to an increased risk of heart disease.

Some examples of healthful fat sources that may be included in the diabetic diet include:
- Avocados: These fruits are high in monounsaturated fats and may be added to salads, sandwiches, or used as a spread in lieu of butter or mayonnaise.

- Nuts and seeds: Almonds, walnuts, flaxseeds, and chia seeds are all wonderful sources of healthful fats. They may be eaten as a snack, added to smoothies or yogurt, or used as toppings for salads and cereals.

- Olive oil: This oil is a mainstay in Mediterranean cuisine and is high in monounsaturated fats. It may be used for cooking, dressing salads, or pouring over roasted vegetables.

- Fatty fish: mackerel, Salmon, and sardines are large in omega-3 fatty acids. Aim to incorporate these fish in your diet at least twice a week.

- Nut butter: Natural nut butter produced from almonds, peanuts, or cashews may be a delightful and healthy addition to the diabetic diet. Just be sure to buy versions without added sweeteners or hydrogenated oils.

Incorporating healthy fats into the diabetic diet is vital for maintaining general health and regulating blood sugar levels. As usual, it is important to speak with a healthcare practitioner or registered dietitian for individualized recommendations on adding healthy fats into your unique diabetes meal plan.

Portion Control and Moderation

Portion management and moderation are crucial factors in maintaining a diabetic diet. These principles encompass recognizing the right quantity of food to ingest and learning self-control when it comes to eating. By practicing portion control and moderation, persons with diabetes may better regulate their blood sugar levels and maintain a healthy weight.

Portion control refers to the practice of consuming certain quantities of food at each meal or snack. It requires being cautious of serving quantities and avoiding overeating. This is crucial for those with diabetes since ingesting too much food, even if it is healthful, may contribute to high blood sugar levels. By reducing portion sizes, people may better regulate their carbohydrate consumption, which directly influences blood sugar levels.

One technique to practice portion management is by using measuring cups, spoons, or a food scale to correctly measure meal servings. This may be particularly useful when it comes to carbs, since they have the most substantial influence on blood sugar levels. For example, a portion of carbs is normally approximately 15 grams, therefore calculating out this amount may assist patients with diabetes maintain better blood sugar management.

Another part of portion management is being attentive of the sorts of meals ingested. It is vital to incorporate a range of nutrient-dense foods, such as fruits, vegetables, lean meats, and whole grains, while also being conscious of their portion amounts. By concentrating on these sorts of meals, folks may feel filled while yet maintaining stable blood sugar levels.

Moderation goes hand in hand with portion management and entails eating a balanced range of meals in reasonable proportions. It implies not denying oneself of beloved meals but rather enjoying them in moderation. For those with diabetes, this may mean savoring a tiny piece of cake on a special occasion or having a modest scoop of ice cream sometimes.

Moderation also pertains to the frequency of consuming particular meals. For example, meals that are heavy in saturated fats or added sugars should be taken sparingly. These include fried meals, sweet desserts, and processed snacks. By restricting the consumption of certain items, people may maintain better blood sugar control and lower the risk of problems linked with diabetes.

Practicing portion control and moderation may be tough, particularly in a world where enormous quantities and decadent meals are easily accessible. However, there are techniques that may help persons with diabetes apply these ideas into their everyday life. These include:

- Planning meals and snacks in advance: By planning ahead, people may ensure they have proper portion sizes and balanced meals accessible. This may help avoid impulsive or excessive eating.

- Using smaller plates and bowls: Research has shown that using smaller plates and bowls might mislead the mind into feeling satiated with fewer servings. This might be particularly useful for persons with diabetes who may struggle with portion management.

- Eating mindfully: Paying attention to hunger and fullness signals might help persons with diabetes better judge proper meal sizes. Eating deliberately, appreciating each mouthful, and being present throughout meals may also help reduce overeating.

- Seeking assistance: Joining a support group or working with a qualified dietitian may give direction and accountability when it comes to portion management and moderation. These specialists may assist consumers build tailored meal plans and suggest solutions for controlling portion sizes.

Portion management and moderation are crucial elements in maintaining a diabetic diet. By adopting portion management, persons with diabetes may better regulate their blood sugar levels by ingesting proper quantities of food, particularly carbs. Moderation entails eating a balanced range of meals in reasonable proportions, while yet allowing for occasional excesses. By implementing these ideas into their everyday lives, persons with diabetes may maintain stable blood sugar levels, attain a healthy weight, and enhance overall well-being.

Fiber and its Benefits for Diabetic Patients

Importance of Dietary Fiber in Diabetes Management

Dietary fiber has a critical function in the control of diabetes. It is a form of carbohydrate that is not broken down by the body and hence does not substantially elevate blood sugar levels. Instead, insulin passes through the digestive system substantially intact, giving various health advantages for those with diabetes.

One of the key advantages of dietary fiber is its ability to help manage blood sugar levels. When ingested, fiber slows down the absorption of glucose into the circulation, reducing fast rises in blood sugar after meals. This may be especially advantageous for persons with diabetes who need to maintain their blood sugar levels to prevent problems.

In addition to its influence on blood sugar regulation, dietary fiber also benefits in weight management. High-fiber meals tend to be more filling and take longer to digest, which may help folks feel full and reduce overeating. This may be particularly essential for those with diabetes who commonly struggle with weight management since excess weight can lead to insulin resistance and poor blood sugar control.

Furthermore, dietary fiber plays a critical function in improving digestive health. It provides volume to the stool, avoiding constipation and facilitating regular bowel motions. This may be especially advantageous for those with diabetes who may develop gastrointestinal difficulties as a consequence of their disease or certain drugs.

Another key advantage of dietary fiber is its influence on heart health. High-fiber meals, such as whole grains, legumes, fruits, and vegetables, have been demonstrated to lessen the risk of heart disease, which is a major consequence of diabetes. Fiber helps decrease cholesterol levels by adhering to cholesterol in the digestive tract and inhibiting its absorption into the circulation.

To include more dietary fiber into a diabetic diet, it is crucial to concentrate on eating a range of high-fiber foods. These include whole grains like oats, brown rice, and quinoa, legumes such as beans and lentils, fruits and vegetables (particularly those with edible skins or seeds), and nuts and seeds. It is vital to highlight that increasing fiber intake should be done gradually and accompanied by enough hydration intake to minimize stomach discomfort.

Dietary fiber has a key role in the control of diabetes. It helps balance blood sugar levels, assists in weight management, supports digestive health, and decreases the risk of heart disease. By including high-fiber foods into their diet, persons with diabetes may enhance their overall health and well-being. It is vital to check with a healthcare expert or registered dietitian to establish the proper quantity of dietary fiber for individual requirements and to provide a well-balanced and healthy diet.

High-Fiber Food Choices

As a diabetic, it is crucial to select healthy dietary choices that are rich in fiber. Fiber is a form of carbohydrate that is not digested by the body, which means it does not boost blood sugar levels. Instead, fiber helps to control blood sugar levels and may also enhance cholesterol levels and digestion.

There are several high-fiber food selections that are appropriate for a diabetic diet. Some examples include entire grains, such as brown rice, quinoa, and whole wheat bread. These foods are rich in fiber and also include key nutrients like vitamins and minerals.

Vegetables are also a wonderful source of fiber. Leafy greens like spinach and kale, as well as cruciferous veggies like broccoli and cauliflower, are all terrific options. These veggies are low in calories and carbs, making them great for diabetics.

Fruits may also be a healthy source of fiber, but it is crucial to pick fruits that are low in sugar. Berries, apples, and pears are all rich in fiber and low in sugar. It is better to avoid fruits like bananas and grapes, which are richer in sugar.

Legumes like beans, lentils, and chickpeas are also rich in fiber and protein. They may be used in a number of cuisines, from soups and stews to salads and dips.

A diabetic diet should concentrate on whole, unprocessed foods that are rich in fiber and low in sugar. By choosing these smart meal choices, diabetics may improve their blood sugar management and general health.

Increasing Fiber Intake Safely

Increasing fiber intake properly is a significant factor for those with diabetes. Fiber is a form of carbohydrate that is not digested by the body, which means it does not boost blood sugar levels. Instead, fiber helps to control blood sugar levels and may also enhance cholesterol levels and digestion.

There are several high-fiber food selections that are appropriate for a diabetic diet. Whole grains, such as brown rice, quinoa, and whole wheat bread, are good sources of fiber and also include key elements including vitamins and minerals. Vegetables like spinach, kale, broccoli, and cauliflower are also rich in fiber and low in calories and carbs, making them great for diabetics.

Fruits may also be a healthy source of fiber, but it is crucial to pick fruits that are low in sugar. Berries, apples, and pears are all rich in fiber and low in sugar. It is better to avoid fruits like bananas and grapes, which are richer in sugar.

Legumes like beans, lentils, and chickpeas are also rich in fiber and protein. They may be used in a number of cuisines, from soups and stews to salads and dips.

When increasing fiber consumption, it is vital to do so gradually to prevent digestive difficulties like bloating and gas. It is advisable to increase fiber intake by 5 grams each day until reaching the required quantity.

Increasing fiber intake safely is an essential concern for patients with diabetes. By eating whole, unprocessed meals that are rich in fiber and low in sugar, diabetics may improve their blood sugar management and general health.

Cooking Techniques and Tips for Diabetic-Friendly Meals

Healthy Cooking Methods for Diabetic Patients

Cooking procedures have a vital impact on the health of those with diabetes. Unhealthy cooking practices may raise the risk of heart disease, which is already greater in those with diabetes. However, good cooking techniques may assist to enhance blood sugar management and general health.

One of the healthiest cooking techniques for diabetics is steaming. Steaming vegetables, fish, and chicken helps to keep their nutrition and taste without adding any additional fat or calories. It is also a fast and simple cooking technique that does not need any extra oil or butter.

Grilling is another healthy cooking option for diabetes. Grilling meats and vegetables enables excess fat to drain away, lowering calorie and fat consumption. However, it is vital to prevent charring or burning the food, since this might contain toxic substances that raise the risk of cancer.

Baking and roasting are other healthful cooking options for diabetes. These techniques do not need any extra fat or oil and may be used for a range of meals, from vegetables to lean meats like chicken and fish.

Stir-frying is a healthy cooking technique for diabetes as long as it is done with minimum oil and lots of veggies. This approach provides for rapid cooking and keeps the nutrients in the veggies.

Boiling is a healthy cooking technique for diabetes when used for vegetables and whole grains. However, it is vital to avoid cooking items like pasta and potatoes for too long, since this might raise their glycemic index.

Proper cooking practices are vital for those with diabetes. Steaming, grilling, baking, roasting, stir-frying, and boiling are all healthy cooking techniques that may assist to enhance blood sugar management and general health. It is crucial to avoid unhealthy cooking techniques like deep-frying and using excessive quantities of oil or butter.

Grilling and Roasting

Grilling and roasting are cooking techniques that might be useful for persons following a diabetic diet. These techniques include cooking food at high temperatures without the need for extra fats or oils, making them a healthier alternative compared to frying or sautéing.

When it comes to grilling, it entails cooking food directly on a grill or barbecue over an open flame or heat source. This approach permits excess fats to drain out from the dish, resulting in a decreased total fat level. For persons with diabetes, this may be useful since it helps to minimize the consumption of harmful fats that can lead to weight gain and poor blood sugar management.

Grilling also helps to keep the natural tastes of the food, making it an enticing alternative for people trying to improve the taste of their meals without depending on additional sweeteners or sauces. This is especially essential for those with diabetes who need to watch their sugar consumption and avoid excessive usage of condiments that may contain hidden sugars.

Roasting, on the other hand, entails cooking food in an oven at high temperatures. This approach is widely used for vegetables, meats, and poultry. Similar to grilling, roasting needs minimum additional fats or oils, making it a healthier cooking alternative. It lets the natural tastes of the food to grow and increase, resulting in tasty and healthy meals.

Roasting veggies may be an excellent method to integrate extra fiber into a diabetic diet. Vegetables like broccoli, cauliflower, Brussels sprouts, and sweet potatoes may be roasted to perfection, delivering a range of important nutrients and nutritional fiber. Roasted meats and poultry may also be eaten in moderation as part of a balanced diabetic diet, as long as lean cuts are selected and extra fat is reduced.

Both grilling and roasting provide the benefit of being diverse cooking techniques. A large variety of meals may be cooked using these approaches, enabling those with diabetes to enjoy a diversified and tasty diet. It is vital, however, to be cautious of portion proportions and to prevent overcooking or charring the food, since this may lead to the development of potentially hazardous substances.

Grilling and roasting are cooking methods that can be beneficial for individuals following a diabetic diet. They enable the production of tasty and healthy meals with little extra fats or oils. By including grilled or roasted items into their diet, persons with diabetes may enjoy gourmet meals while maintaining excellent blood sugar management and general health. As always, it is crucial to check with a healthcare expert or registered dietitian for customized nutritional guidance and recommendations.

Steaming and Boiling

Steaming and boiling are two cooking procedures that might potentially be advantageous for persons following a diabetic diet. These techniques include cooking food using water or steam, without the need for extra fats or oils. When it comes to steaming, it entails preparing food by exposing it to steam. This delicate cooking technique helps to keep the original tastes, colors, and nutrients of the food. Steaming is especially good for vegetables, since it helps to retain their texture and nutritious content. Vegetables such as broccoli, carrots, and green beans may be steamed to perfection, offering a great supply of vitamins, minerals, and nutritional fiber.

Steaming is favorable for those with diabetes since it does not entail the use of additional fats or oils. This implies that steamed meals are fewer in calories and harmful fats, which may lead to weight gain and poor blood sugar management. Steaming also helps to retain the integrity of the food's natural sugars, making it an ideal cooking technique for persons who need to regulate their sugar consumption. Boiling, on the other hand, includes cooking food in boiling water. This technique is often used for pasta, grains, and legumes. Boiling may assist to soften certain meals and make them simpler to digest. It is vital, however, to be aware of the cooking time, since overcooking might lead to a loss of nutrients.

When boiling vegetables or starchy meals such as potatoes or rice, it is advisable to use minimum quantities of water and prevent prolonged boiling durations. This helps to avoid the leaching of nutrients into the water. Additionally, it is suggested to take the cooking water as part of the meal, since it may include some of the water-soluble vitamins and minerals. Both steaming and boiling provide the benefit of being easy and convenient cooking procedures. They need minimum preparation and equipment, making them perfect for persons with hectic lives.

Furthermore, these approaches allow for the preparation of a broad range of meals, offering patients with diabetes the option to enjoy a diversified and healthy diet.

Steaming and boiling are cooking techniques that might be useful for persons following a diabetic diet. They include cooking food using water or steam, without the need for extra fats or oils. By including steamed or boiled items into their diet, persons with diabetes may enjoy gourmet meals while maintaining excellent blood sugar management and general health. As always, it is crucial to check with a healthcare expert or registered dietitian for customized nutritional guidance and recommendations.

Stir-Frying and Sautéing

Stir-frying and sautéing are two cooking techniques that might also be advantageous for persons following a diabetic diet. These techniques include cooking food fast in a minimal quantity of oil or fat, resulting in tasty and healthful meals. When it comes to stir-frying, it includes heating bite-sized bits of food in a hot skillet or wok with a tiny quantity of oil. This approach allows for rapid cooking, keeping the inherent aromas, colors, and nutrients of the food. Stir-frying is especially good for vegetables, lean meats, and seafood.

Stir-frying is good for those with diabetes since it takes just a minimal quantity of oil or fat. This implies that stir-fried foods are fewer in calories and bad fats compared to other cooking techniques that may need more oil. By using moderate quantities of oil, folks may still enjoy delectable meals while keeping optimal blood sugar management.

Sautéing, on the other hand, entails cooking food rapidly in a minimal quantity of oil or fat over medium to high heat. This technique is widely used for browning or searing foods such as meats, poultry, and fish. Sautéing helps to generate rich tastes and textures in the food, making it a popular cooking technique for numerous cuisines.

Stir-frying and sautéing are cooking techniques that may be useful for persons following a diabetic diet. They entail cooking food rapidly in a tiny quantity of oil or fat, resulting in tasty and healthful meals. By including stir-fried or sautéed meals into their diet, persons with diabetes may have a variety.

Reducing Added Sugars in Recipes

Natural Sweeteners Substitutes

Natural sweeteners may be a beneficial option for persons following a diabetic diet. These sweeteners give a means to satisfy a sweet appetite without producing large rises in blood sugar levels. By selecting natural sweeteners, patients with diabetes may enjoy the taste of sweetness while maintaining appropriate blood sugar control. One popular natural sweetener alternative is stevia. Stevia is extracted from the leaves of the Stevia rebaudiana plant and is recognized for its extreme sweetness. It has zero calories and does not elevate blood sugar levels, making it an acceptable alternative for persons with diabetes. Stevia may be used in a range of dishes, including drinks, baked products, and desserts.

Another natural sweetener replacement is monk fruit extract. Monk fruit extract is extracted from the monk fruit, also known as Luo Han Guo. It is substantially sweeter than sugar yet has o calories and does not impact blood sugar levels. Monk fruit extract may be used in a similar manner as sugar and can be added to drinks, sauces, and baked products. Xylitol is another natural sweetener that may be used as a replacement for sugar. It is generated from the fibrous sections of plants and has a comparable taste to sugar. Xylitol has less calories than sugar and has a low influence on blood sugar levels, making it acceptable for those with diabetes. It may be used in baking, cooking, and as a sweetener for drinks.

Erythritol is a sugar alcohol that is naturally present in fruits and fermented foods. It has a similar flavor to sugar but has less calories and has a minor impact on blood sugar levels. Erythritol may be used in a number of recipes and can be replaced for sugar at a 1:1 ratio. When utilizing natural sweeteners as alternatives for sugar, it is crucial to realize that they might still add to total calorie consumption. While they may not spike blood sugar levels as drastically as sugar, ingesting excessive quantities of natural sweeteners may still have an influence on weight management and general health. It is vital to utilize natural sweeteners in moderation and to evaluate the entire composition of the meal or preparation.

Natural sweeteners may be a beneficial option for persons following a diabetic diet. Options such as stevia, monk fruit extract, xylitol, and erythritol give sweetness without generating large rises in blood sugar levels. By including these natural sweeteners into their diet, persons with diabetes may enjoy the taste of sweetness while maintaining appropriate blood sugar control. As always, it is crucial to check with a healthcare expert or registered dietitian for customized nutritional guidance and recommendations.

Reading Food Labels for Hidden Sugars

Reading food labels for hidden sugars is vital for persons following a diabetic diet. While natural sweeteners may be a helpful replacement for sugar, it is still vital to be cautious of hidden sugars in processed foods. These hidden sugars may induce surges in blood sugar levels and prevent proper blood sugar management.

When reading food labels, it is vital to check for distinct designations that indicate the presence of added sugars. Some popular names for added sugars include sucrose, glucose, fructose, corn syrup, and high-fructose corn syrup. These sugars may be found in numerous forms, such as syrups, nectars, and concentrates. Another useful tool when reading food labels is the nutrition information panel. This panel offers information on the quantity of total carbs and sugars in a serving of the product. It is vital to remember that the total carbs comprise both naturally occurring and added sugars. By comparing the quantity of total carbs to the serving size, consumers may establish how much sugar is in each dish.

By being aware of the numerous names for added sugars, paying attention to the sequence of ingredients, and examining the nutrition information panel, consumers may make educated decisions regarding their food consumption. It is always advisable to check with a healthcare practitioner or certified dietitian for specific information on reading food labels and managing a diabetic diet.

Strategies for Cutting Down on Added Sugars

Cutting down on added sugars is vital for persons following a diabetic diet in order to maintain appropriate blood sugar control. Here are some techniques to help limit the intake of added sugars:

1. Choose whole, unprocessed foods: Opt for fresh fruits, vegetables, lean meats, and whole grains instead than processed meals. These whole foods

are naturally low in added sugars and include key nutrients that may help regulate blood sugar levels.

2. Read food labels: When buying packaged goods, reading food labels is vital. Look for other names that indicate the presence of added sugars, such as sucrose, glucose, fructose, corn syrup, and high-fructose corn syrup. Avoid items that have added sugars stated towards the top of the ingredient list, since this signals a substantial quantity of added sugars.

3. Be cautious of portion proportions: Even if a product is labeled as "sugar-free" or "no added sugars," it is crucial to be mindful of portion amounts. Consuming significant amounts of these items might still alter blood sugar levels owing to the inclusion of natural sweeteners or sugar alcohols. Stick to suggested serving portions and check blood sugar levels appropriately.

4. Limit sugary drinks: Sugary beverages including soda, fruit juices, and sweetened teas may contribute a considerable quantity of additional sugars to the diet. Opt for water, unsweetened tea, or flavored water with no added sweeteners instead. If seeking something sweet, try infusing water with

fruits or adding a dash of lemon or lime juice for taste.

5. consider healthier choices: Instead of reaching for sugary snacks and sweets, consider healthier alternatives. For example, go for fresh fruit or unsweetened yogurt instead of sweets or candies. Use natural sweeteners like stevia or monk fruit extract in moderation as a replacement for sugar.

6. Cook at home: By making meals at home, consumers have better control over the items used and may prevent hidden sweets. Experiment with herbs, spices, and natural flavorings to improve the taste of foods without depending on added sugars.

7. Seek support: It might be tough to cut down on added sugars alone. Seek help from healthcare experts, licensed dietitians, or support groups to gain direction, recommendations, and inspiration. They may give tailored guidance and solutions for managing a diabetic diet while lowering additional sugar consumption.

Diabetic–Friendly Recipes and Meal Plan

Breakfast Recipes

Breakfast is typically considered the most essential meal of the day, particularly for persons following a diabetic diet. A well-balanced breakfast may help normalize blood sugar levels and give consistent energy throughout the day. Here are some breakfast dishes that are good for a diabetic diet:

1. Veggie Omelet: Whisk up two eggs and add a variety of chopped veggies such as bell peppers, spinach, mushrooms, and onions. Cook the mixture in a non-stick pan with a little olive oil until the eggs are set. Serve with a side of whole grain bread or a small quantity of cooked quinoa.

2. Greek Yogurt Parfait: Layer plain Greek yogurt with fresh berries, such as strawberries, blueberries, or raspberries, in a glass or dish. Top with a sprinkling of chopped nuts, such as almonds or walnuts, and a drizzle of sugar-free honey or a sprinkle of cinnamon for extra flavor.

3. Overnight Chia Pudding: Mix together 1/4 cup of chia seeds with 1 cup of unsweetened almond milk

or coconut milk in a container. Add a few drops of vanilla essence and a sprinkle of cinnamon for taste. Let it lie in the refrigerator overnight to enable the chia seeds to absorb the liquid and produce a pudding-like consistency. Serve with a handful of fresh berries on top.

4. Whole Grain Pancakes: Make pancakes using whole grain flour or a blend of whole wheat flour and almond flour. Add mashed bananas or unsweetened applesauce to the batter for natural sweetness instead of sugar. Top with a dollop of Greek yogurt and a sprinkling of cinnamon.

5. Avocado Toast: Toast a piece of whole grain bread and put mashed avocado on top. Sprinkle with salt, pepper, and a squeeze of lemon juice. For extra protein, top with a poached egg or a piece of smoked salmon.

6. Vegetable Frittata: Sautee a variety of vegetables, such as zucchini, bell peppers, onions, and spinach, in a non-stick skillet with a little olive oil. Whisk together four eggs with a splash of milk and pour over the veggies. Cook until the eggs are set then sprinkle with shredded cheese, such as feta or Parmesan. Serve with a side of whole grain bread.

7. Smoothie Bowl: Blend together a variety of frozen berries, spinach or kale, unsweetened almond milk or coconut milk, and a scoop of protein powder or Greek yogurt for additional protein. Pour the mixture into a bowl and top with sliced almonds, chia seeds, and a sprinkling of unsweetened coconut flakes.

Remember to speak with a healthcare expert or certified dietitian for specialized information on breakfast recipes and maintaining a diabetic diet. They may give customized advice based on individual health requirements and objectives.

High-Fiber Breakfast Options

High-fiber breakfast alternatives are especially advantageous for persons following a diabetic diet. Fiber is a form of carbohydrate that is not digested by the body, meaning it does not boost blood sugar levels. Instead, it travels through the digestive system, offering several health advantages.

One of the key advantages of having high-fiber meals for breakfast is that they help balance blood sugar levels. When combined with carbs, fiber slows down the absorption of glucose into the circulation, avoiding rises in blood sugar levels. This is particularly critical for those with diabetes, since maintaining blood sugar levels is key for treating the illness.

Additionally, high-fiber breakfast alternatives create a sensation of fullness and may aid with weight control. Fiber-rich meals take longer to digest, improving fullness and lowering the probability of overeating later in the day. This may be especially useful for those with diabetes who are also attempting to reduce weight or maintain a healthy weight.

Furthermore, a diet rich in fiber has been related with a lower risk of heart disease. Soluble fiber, present in foods such as oats, barley, and legumes, has been demonstrated to reduce cholesterol levels. By integrating high-fiber breakfast alternatives into their diet, persons with diabetes may enhance their heart health and minimize their risk of cardiovascular problems.

Some examples of high-fiber breakfast items suited for a diabetic diet include:
1. Overnight oats: Combine rolled oats with unsweetened almond milk or Greek yogurt and let it lie in the refrigerator overnight. In the morning, add toppings such as fresh berries, chopped nuts,

and a drizzle of sugar-free honey or a sprinkle of cinnamon.

2. Whole grain cereal: Choose a cereal that is rich in fiber and low in added sugars. Look for alternatives that have at least 5 grams of fiber per serving and avoid those with added sugars or artificial sweeteners. Serve with unsweetened almond milk or Greek yogurt and top with sliced fruit.

3. Bran muffins: Make homemade muffins using healthy wheat flour and bran. Add in vegetables like as shredded carrots or zucchini, chopped almonds, and dried fruits for extra taste and fiber. Be aware of portion proportions and avoid adding excessive quantities of sugar or harmful fats.

4. Chia seed pudding: Mix together chia seeds with unsweetened almond milk or coconut milk and let it rest in the refrigerator until it thickens. Add flavorings such as vanilla essence or chocolate powder and top with fresh berries or sliced almonds.

5. Whole grain toast with nut butter: Choose whole grain bread that is rich in fiber and cover it with a natural nut butter, such as almond or peanut

butter. Top with sliced banana or berries for extra nutrition and taste.

Incorporating high-fiber breakfast alternatives into a diabetic diet may have various health advantages, including better blood sugar management, enhanced satiety, and lower risk of heart disease. It is vital to speak with a healthcare expert or registered dietitian for specific counsel on adding fiber into a diabetic diet, since individual requirements may differ.

Low-Carb and Protein-Rich Breakfasts

Low-carb and protein-rich breakfasts may be good for persons following a diabetic diet. These breakfast alternatives may help balance blood sugar levels, enhance fullness, and assist weight control.

One of the primary benefits of having low-carb breakfasts for those with diabetes is that they may help manage blood sugar levels. Carbohydrates are the key food that impacts blood sugar levels, therefore limiting carb consumption helps reduce rises in glucose. By choosing for low-carb breakfasts, consumers may avoid the quick increase and fall of blood sugar that can occur with high-carb meals. This is especially crucial for those with diabetes who need to carefully monitor their blood sugar levels.

Additionally, protein-rich breakfasts may enhance fullness and help reduce hunger throughout the day. Protein takes longer to digest than carbs, which means it might keep you feeling full for longer times. This may be good for those with diabetes who are attempting to maintain their weight or lose weight, since it can lower the risk of overeating or nibbling on unhealthy foods later in the day.

Furthermore, protein-rich meals may help muscular health and maintenance. Diabetes may increase the risk of muscle loss and impaired muscular function, thus keeping an appropriate intake of protein is vital. Including protein-rich meals in breakfast, such as eggs, Greek yogurt, or lean meats, may assist deliver the required amino acids for muscle repair and development.

Some examples of low-carb and protein-rich breakfast alternatives acceptable for a diabetic diet include:

1. Veggie omelet: Whisk together eggs or egg whites with chopped veggies such as spinach, bell peppers, and mushrooms. Cook in a non-stick pan with a

tiny bit of olive oil or cooking spray. Serve with a side of avocado or a piece of whole grain bread.

2. Greek yogurt with nuts and seeds: Choose plain Greek yogurt and top it with a handful of mixed nuts and seeds, such as almonds, walnuts, chia seeds, and flaxseeds. Add a sprinkle of cinnamon or a drop of sugar-free honey for extra taste.

3. Smoked salmon roll-ups: Roll up slices of smoked salmon with a topping of cream cheese or avocado. Add some sliced cucumber or tomato for freshness and serve with a side of mixed greens or a small serving of low-carb veggies.

4. Protein smoothie: Blend together unsweetened almond milk or coconut milk with a scoop of protein powder, a handful of spinach or kale, and a small quantity of low-glycemic fruits such as berries or half a banana. Optional ingredients include nut butter, chia seeds, or flaxseeds for extra protein and fiber.

5. Cottage cheese with berries: Enjoy a dish of cottage cheese with a handful of fresh berries, such as strawberries, blueberries, or raspberries. Sprinkle a little cinnamon or drizzle with sugar-free honey for extra sweetness.

Incorporating low-carb and protein-rich breakfast alternatives into a diabetic diet may give various advantages, including better blood sugar management, enhanced satiety, and support for muscle function. It is vital to speak with a healthcare practitioner or registered dietitian for specific advice on integrating these breakfast alternatives into a diabetic diet, since individual requirements may differ.

Quick and Easy Breakfast Ideas

Quick and simple breakfast ideas for a diabetic diet may give those with diabetes with healthy and delicious alternatives to start their day. These meals are meant to help balance blood sugar levels, enhance satiety, and assist weight control.

One of the primary benefits of these breakfast options is that they are low in carbs. Carbohydrates have the most influence on blood sugar levels, thus limiting their consumption helps minimize rises in glucose. By choosing for low-carb breakfasts, consumers may avoid the quick increase and fall of blood sugar that can occur with high-carb meals. This is especially crucial for those with diabetes who need to carefully monitor their blood sugar levels.

In addition to being low in carbohydrates, these breakfast alternatives are also high in protein. Protein takes longer to digest than carbs, which means it might keep you feeling full for longer times. This may be good for those with diabetes who are attempting to maintain their weight or lose weight, since it can lower the risk of overeating or nibbling on unhealthy foods later in the day.

Furthermore, protein-rich meals may help muscular health and maintenance. Diabetes may increase the risk of muscle loss and impaired muscular function, thus keeping an appropriate intake of protein is vital. Including protein-rich meals in breakfast, such as eggs, Greek yogurt, or lean meats, may assist deliver the required amino acids for muscle repair and development.

Here are some quick and simple breakfast alternatives acceptable for a diabetic diet:

1. Veggie omelet: Whisk together eggs or egg whites with chopped veggies such as spinach, bell peppers, and mushrooms. Cook in a non-stick pan with a tiny bit of olive oil or cooking spray. Serve with a side of avocado or a piece of whole grain bread.

2. Greek yogurt with nuts and seeds: Choose plain Greek yogurt and top it with a handful of mixed nuts and seeds, such as almonds, walnuts, chia seeds, and flaxseeds. Add a sprinkle of cinnamon or a drop of sugar-free honey for extra taste.

3. Smoked salmon roll-ups: Roll up slices of smoked salmon with a topping of cream cheese or avocado. Add some sliced cucumber or tomato for freshness and serve with a side of mixed greens or a small serving of low-carb veggies.

4. Protein smoothie: Blend together unsweetened almond milk or coconut milk with a scoop of protein powder, a handful of spinach or kale, and a small quantity of low-glycemic fruits such as berries or half a banana. Optional ingredients include nut butter, chia seeds, or flaxseeds for extra protein and fiber.

5. Cottage cheese with berries: Enjoy a dish of cottage cheese with a handful of fresh berries, such as strawberries, blueberries, or raspberries. Sprinkle a little cinnamon or drizzle with sugar-free honey for extra sweetness.

Combining these quick and easy breakfast ideas into a diabetic diet can supply several benefits, containing improved blood sugar control, improved satiety, and support for muscle health. It is crucial to consult with a healthcare professional or registered dietitian for personalized recommendations on incorporating these breakfast choices into a diabetic diet, as personal appetites may vary.

Lunch Recipes

Balanced Lunches with a Variety of Nutrients

Balanced meals with a range of nutrients are necessary for persons following a diabetic diet. These meals should concentrate on including a balance of carbs, proteins, and healthy fats to give sustained energy, induce satiety, and support overall health.

When preparing a balanced lunch for a diabetic diet, it is vital to consider the glycemic index (GI) of the items selected. The glycemic index assesses how rapidly carbohydrates in diet elevate blood sugar levels. Those with a high GI may induce a quick surge in blood sugar, whereas those with a low GI have a slower and more progressive influence on blood sugar levels. Choosing meals with a low or moderate GI may help persons with diabetes regulate their blood sugar levels more efficiently.

Here are some suggestions for balanced meals with a range of nutrients for a diabetic diet:
1. Grilled chicken salad: Start with a bed of mixed greens and add grilled chicken breast, cherry tomatoes, cucumber slices, and avocado. Top with a

sprinkling of feta cheese or a handful of almonds for extra flavor and healthy fats. Dress the salad with a simple vinaigrette prepared from olive oil, vinegar, and herbs.

2. Quinoa and vegetable stir-fry: Cook quinoa according to package directions and put aside. In a non-stick skillet, sauté an array of bright veggies such as bell peppers, broccoli, carrots, and snap peas. Add cooked quinoa and mix together with a low-sodium soy sauce or a sprinkle of olive oil and lemon juice.

3. Turkey lettuce wraps: Use big lettuce leaves as a replacement for bread or tortillas and fill them with lean turkey pieces, chopped avocado, and tomato. Add some mustard or hummus for added taste. Serve with a side of raw vegetables or a small amount of healthy grain crackers.

4. Lentil soup with whole grain bread: Prepare a hearty lentil soup using low-sodium broth, lentils, onions, carrots, and celery. Season with herbs and spices for extra taste. Pair the soup with a piece of whole grain bread or a small quantity of whole grain crackers for a balanced meal.

5. Baked salmon with roasted vegetables: Season a salmon fillet with herbs, lemon juice, and a splash of olive oil. Bake in the oven until cooked through. Serve with a side of roasted vegetables, such as Brussels sprouts, cauliflower, and sweet potatoes, for a healthy and fulfilling meal.

When designing balanced meals for a diabetic diet, it is crucial to consider portion sizes and the total calorie composition of the meal. It may be good to speak with a healthcare practitioner or registered dietitian for tailored counseling on portion management and meal planning. Additionally, monitoring blood sugar levels and making modifications to the lunch selections may be important to achieve optimum blood sugar management throughout the day.

Balanced meals with a range of nutrients are necessary for persons following a diabetic diet. By ingesting a balance of carbs, proteins, and healthy fats, people may maintain stable blood sugar levels, feel content, and support their overall health. Consulting with a healthcare expert or qualified dietitian is suggested to modify these lunch ideas to specific requirements and maintain optimum treatment of diabetes.

Packable Lunches for Work or School

Packable lunches for work or school may be a practical and healthful choice for persons following a diabetic diet. These meals should concentrate on including a balance of carbs, proteins, and healthy fats to give sustained energy, induce satiety, and support overall health. It is also vital to examine the glycemic index (GI) of the meals selected to assist regulate blood sugar levels properly.

Here are some options for packable lunches for a diabetic diet:

1. Whole grain wrap with lean protein: Use a whole grain wrap or tortilla as a basis and fill it with lean protein such as grilled chicken, turkey, or tofu. Add lots of bright veggies like lettuce, tomatoes, cucumbers, and bell peppers. Include a tiny bit of avocado or hummus for healthy fats. Roll it up firmly and fill it with some raw vegetables or a tiny piece of fruit.

2. Quinoa salad: Cook quinoa according to package directions and let it cool. Mix it with an array of chopped veggies such cherry tomatoes, cucumbers, bell peppers, and red onions. Add some cooked chickpeas or grilled prawns for protein. Dress the salad with a light vinaigrette prepared from olive

oil, lemon juice, and herbs. Pack it in a jar and consume it chilled or at room temperature.

3. Greek yogurt with mixed berries and nuts: Choose a plain Greek yogurt and add a handful of mixed berries like strawberries, blueberries, or raspberries. Sprinkle some crushed nuts such as almonds or walnuts for extra crunch and healthy fats. Pack it in a small container and add a separate serving of good grain crackers or a tiny piece of dark chocolate for a pleasant and balanced meal.

4. Vegetable and lentil soup: Prepare a pot of vegetable and lentil soup using low-sodium broth, onions, carrots, celery, and your choice of veggies. Add cooked lentils for protein and season with herbs and spices for flavor. Divide the soup into separate containers and wrap them with a side of whole grain bread or a small quantity of whole grain crackers.

5. Salad in a jar: Layer a mason jar with your favorite salad components, beginning with the dressing at the bottom, followed by firm veggies like cucumbers or bell peppers, then protein such as grilled chicken or tofu, and lastly lush greens. Seal the jar firmly and refrigerate it until ready to

consume. Shake the container to blend the contents before eating a fresh and crisp salad.

When making packable lunches for a diabetic diet, it is vital to consider portion sizes and the total calorie composition of the meal. It may be beneficial to use measuring cups or a food scale to ensure correct portioning. Additionally, monitoring blood sugar levels and making modifications to the lunch selections may be important to maintain optimum blood sugar management throughout the day.

Packable lunches for work or school might be a handy and healthful choice for persons following a diabetic diet. By ingesting a balance of carbs, proteins, and healthy fats, people may maintain stable blood sugar levels, feel content, and support their overall health. It is vital to examine the glycemic index of the foods selected and speak with a healthcare expert or registered dietitian for tailored recommendations on portion management and meal planning.

Salads, Wraps, and Sandwiches

Salads, wraps, and sandwiches may be fantastic alternatives for persons following a diabetic diet since they can offer a balanced mix of nutrients while being simple and quick to carry for work or school. These meals may be adjusted to contain a range of products that are low in glycemic index and rich in fiber, protein, and healthy fats to help regulate blood sugar levels successfully.

Salads are a diverse choice that may be filled with a variety of veggies, lean meats, and healthy fats. Opt for leafy greens like spinach or kale as a basis and add colorful veggies like tomatoes, cucumbers, bell peppers, and carrots. Include a lean protein source such as grilled chicken, turkey, or tofu. To add healthy fats, incorporate alternatives like avocado slices, almonds, or seeds. Avoid high-sugar dressings and instead for homemade dressings prepared with olive oil, lemon juice, and herbs.

Wraps and sandwiches may also be made diabetes-friendly by using whole grain wraps or bread. Choose whole grain choices over refined grains to guarantee a slower release of glucose into the system. Fill the wrap or sandwich with lean proteins such as grilled chicken, turkey, or fish. Add lots of veggies like lettuce, tomatoes, cucumbers, and bell peppers for extra fiber and minerals. Incorporate a modest quantity of healthy fats like avocado or hummus for satiety and taste.

When making these meals, it is crucial to consider portion sizes and the total calorie content. It may be beneficial to use measuring cups or a food scale to ensure correct portioning. Additionally, monitoring blood sugar levels and making modifications to the components used may be important to maintain optimum blood sugar management throughout the day.

Salads, wraps, and sandwiches may be good alternatives for persons following a diabetic diet. By adding a combination of low glycemic index carbs, lean proteins, and healthy fats, these meals may deliver sustained energy, induce satiety, and support overall health. It is necessary to contact a healthcare expert or registered dietitian for tailored counseling on portion restriction and meal planning to achieve the optimum management of blood sugar levels.

Dinner Recipes

Flavorful and Diabetic-Friendly Main Dishes

When following a diabetic diet, it is crucial to pick major meals that are not only tasty but also assist maintain stable blood sugar levels. By adding a variety of tastes and ingredients, consumers may enjoy a varied range of meals while still controlling their diabetes properly. One choice for a tasty and diabetic-friendly main meal is grilled or baked lean meats such as chicken, turkey, or fish. These proteins are low in fat and supply important nutrients without generating rises in blood sugar levels. To improve the taste, marinate the meats with herbs, spices, and citrus juices instead of using sweet marinades or sauces.

Vegetarian choices may also be tasty and acceptable for a diabetic diet. Incorporating plant-based proteins like tofu or tempeh may produce a filling and tasty main meal. These proteins may be marinated or seasoned with herbs and spices to enhance depth of flavor. Additionally, legumes such as lentils, chickpeas, or black beans may be used as a basis for vegetarian main meals, giving both protein and fiber to help balance blood sugar levels.

Incorporating a variety of veggies into major meals is vital for a diabetic diet. Vegetables are low in calories and carbs while being rich in fiber and important minerals. Roasting or stir-frying veggies with herbs, spices, and a tiny quantity of heart-healthy oils like olive oil may enhance their natural tastes. This may be coupled with lean meats or nutritious grains for a balanced and delicious main meal.

Whole grains such as quinoa, brown rice, or whole wheat pasta may be used as a basis for major meals. These grains have a lower glycemic index compared to refined grains, meaning they are digested more slowly and do not produce sudden rises in blood sugar levels. Pairing healthy grains with lean meats and veggies may make a full and nutritious main meal. When making diabetic-friendly main courses, it is crucial to avoid using excessive quantities of salt, sugar, and harmful fats. Instead, depend on herbs, spices, and natural tastes to improve the taste of the food. It is crucial to contact a healthcare practitioner or registered dietitian for specific help on meal planning and quantity management. They may give tailored advice based on unique dietary requirements and objectives. By including savory and diabetes-friendly main dishes into a diabetic diet, patients may maintain stable blood sugar levels while still enjoying great and gratifying meals.

Vegetarian and Vegan Dinner Options

Vegetarian and vegan supper alternatives might be wonderful choices for persons following a diabetic diet. These plant-based meals may offer a diverse variety of tastes, textures, and minerals while helping to maintain stable blood sugar levels. One option for a vegetarian or vegan meal is a substantial salad. Start with a foundation of leafy greens such as spinach or kale, and then add a range of bright veggies including bell peppers, tomatoes, cucumbers, and carrots. To increase protein, add items like tofu, tempeh, or chickpeas. Nuts and seeds may also be added for additional crunch and healthy fats. To enhance the taste, sprinkle the salad with a homemade vinaigrette prepared from olive oil, vinegar, and herbs.

Another alternative is stir-fried veggies with tofu or tempeh. This meal may be produced by sautéing a variety of veggies including broccoli, bell peppers, mushrooms, and snap peas in a modest quantity of heart-healthy oil. Add in cubed tofu or tempeh for protein and season with herbs, spices, and low-sodium soy sauce or tamari. Serve it over a bed of brown rice or quinoa for a full and fulfilling dinner.

For a warming supper alternative, try creating a vegetable curry. Use a variety of veggies including cauliflower, carrots, peas, and bell peppers, and boil them in a fragrant curry sauce prepared from coconut milk and spices like turmeric, cumin, and coriander. Add in tofu or chickpeas for protein and serve it over brown rice or whole wheat naan bread.

Pasta meals may also be changed to match a diabetic diet. Opt for whole wheat spaghetti and combine it with a variety of veggies including zucchini, eggplant, and cherry tomatoes. Instead of using typical tomato sauce, prepare a homemade sauce using roasted red peppers, garlic, and herbs. Top it up with some grated Parmesan cheese or nutritional yeast for extra taste. When cooking vegetarian or vegan dinner alternatives for a diabetic diet, it is crucial to pay attention to portion sizes and the overall balance of macronutrients. Including a source of protein like tofu, tempeh, or beans is vital for balancing blood sugar levels.

Healthy Side Dishes that Complement the Main Course

Healthy side dishes may be a terrific addition to a diabetic diet, as they can give additional nutrients, fiber, and taste to complement the main meal. Here are some ideas for healthful side dishes that are good for persons following a diabetic diet:

1. Roasted veggies: Roasting veggies brings out their inherent sweetness and adds a lovely caramelized taste. Choose a range of bright veggies including Brussels sprouts, cauliflower, carrots, and sweet potatoes. Toss them with a little quantity of heart-healthy oil, such as olive oil, and season with herbs and spices like rosemary, thyme, or paprika. Roast in the oven until soft and golden brown.

2. Quinoa Salad: Quinoa is a healthy whole grain that is high in protein and fiber. Cook quinoa according to package directions and let it cool. Toss it with diced veggies like cucumbers, cherry tomatoes, bell peppers, and red onions. Add some fresh herbs like parsley or cilantro for added taste. Dress the salad with a light vinaigrette prepared from lemon juice, olive oil, and Dijon mustard.

3. Steamed Broccoli with Garlic: Broccoli is a nutrient-dense vegetable that is low in carbs and rich in fiber. Steam broccoli until it is soft but still brilliant green. In a separate skillet, sauté minced garlic in a tiny quantity of heart-healthy oil until aromatic. Toss the steamed broccoli with the garlic oil and season with salt and pepper to taste.

4. Baked Sweet Potato Fries: Sweet potatoes are an excellent source of fiber and vitamins. Cut sweet potatoes into thin strips to resemble fries. Toss them with a little quantity of heart-healthy oil, such as avocado oil, and season with herbs and spices like cinnamon or paprika.

5. Mixed Greens Salad: A simple mixed greens salad may be a delicious and light side meal. Use a variety of leafy greens including spinach, arugula, and romaine lettuce. Top with sliced cucumbers, cherry tomatoes, and radishes. For extra flavor and crunch, sprinkle with some roasted nuts or seeds, such as almonds or pumpkin seeds. Dress the salad with a light vinaigrette prepared from lemon juice, olive oil, and Dijon mustard.

When picking side dishes for a diabetic diet, it is crucial to consider portion sizes and the overall balance of macronutrients.

Snack and Dessert Recipes

Nutritious Snack Ideas for Diabetic Patients

Snacking may be an essential aspect of treating diabetes, since it helps to maintain blood sugar levels and avoid overeating at mealtimes. However, it is vital for patients with diabetes to pick snacks that are low in carbs and rich in fiber, protein, and healthy fats. Here are some healthful snack options that are good for diabetes patients:

1. Greek Yogurt with Berries: Greek yogurt is a fantastic source of protein and calcium, and it has a reduced carbohydrate content compared to conventional yogurt. Top a serving of Greek yogurt with a handful of fresh berries like strawberries, blueberries, or raspberries. Berries are low in sugar and strong in antioxidants and fiber, making them a good option for diabetes individuals.

2. Veggie Sticks with Hummus: Cut up a variety of colorful veggies including carrots, bell peppers, cucumbers, and celery into sticks. Pair them with a small quantity of hummus for a pleasant and healthy snack. Hummus is produced from chickpeas, which are strong in fiber and protein,

making it a fantastic choice for balancing blood sugar levels.

3. Hard-Boiled Eggs: Hard-boiled eggs are a quick and protein-rich snack that may help keep you full and content. They are low in carbs and include critical minerals such vitamins A, D, and B12. Sprinkle some salt and pepper or add a dash of spicy sauce for more taste.

4. Nuts and Seeds: Nuts and seeds are rich with healthy fats, fiber, and protein, making them a great snack for diabetes people. Choose unsalted kinds like almonds, walnuts, pistachios, or pumpkin seeds. Be aware of portion proportions since nuts and seeds are calorie-dense.

5. Cottage Cheese with Flaxseeds: Cottage cheese is a low-fat dairy product that is abundant in protein and calcium. Top a dollop of cottage cheese with a sprinkle of ground flaxseeds for additional fiber and omega-3 fatty acids. Flaxseeds are also proven to help control blood sugar levels.

6. Avocado Slices on Whole Grain Crackers: Avocado is a nutrient-dense fruit that is high in heart-healthy fats and fiber. Slice half an avocado and put it on top of whole grain crackers. Whole

grain crackers contain complex carbs and extra fiber.

7. Roasted Chickpeas: Roasted chickpeas are a crisp and tasty snack that is packed in fiber and protein. Rinse and drain canned chickpeas, mix them with a tiny quantity of heart-healthy oil, and season with herbs and spices like cumin, paprika, or garlic powder. Roast in the oven until crispy.

8. Cheese and Apple Slices: Pairing a piece of low-fat cheese with apple slices may give a mix of protein, fiber, and natural sugars. Choose a low-fat cheese kind like mozzarella or cheddar, and go for a little apple to keep the carbohydrate amount in line.

Consulting with a healthcare expert or registered dietitian may give individualized advice on snack selections and quantity management to fit specific nutritional requirements and objectives.

Sugar-Free and Low-Carb Desserts

For persons with diabetes, finding sweets that are both sugar-free and low in carbs may be a struggle. However, there are still lots of delectable choices available that may fulfill your sweet taste without creating increases in blood sugar levels. Here are some suggestions for sugar-free and low-carb desserts acceptable for a diabetic diet:

1. Sugar-Free Jello: Sugar-free jello is a favorite dessert choice for individuals managing their sugar consumption. It is minimal in calories and carbs, making it a guilt-free pleasure. You may also add some fresh berries or a dollop of sugar-free whipped cream for added taste.

2. Chia Pudding: Chia pudding is a healthful and adaptable dessert that can be created with little ingredients. Simply combine chia seeds with unsweetened almond milk or coconut milk, and let it lie in the refrigerator overnight to thicken. You may add tastes like vanilla essence, cocoa powder, or cinnamon for diversity.

3. Sugar-Free Ice Cream: Many manufacturers now offer sugar-free ice cream alternatives that are sweetened with artificial sweeteners like stevia or erythritol. Look for products that are low in carbs and manufactured with natural ingredients. You may also create your own sugar-free ice cream at home using heavy cream, unsweetened almond milk, and a low-carb sweetener.

4. Dark Chocolate: Dark chocolate with a high proportion of cocoa (70% or above) is lower in sugar and carbs compared to milk chocolate. Enjoy a little piece of dark chocolate as an occasional pleasure. You may also add some nuts or nut butter for extra texture and taste.

5. Sugar-Free Cheesecake: Traditional cheesecake is frequently rich in sugar and carbs, but you can prepare a diabetic-friendly version by using sugar replacements like stevia or erythritol instead. You may also use almond flour or crushed almonds for the crust to lower the carbohydrate load.

6. Berry Parfait: Layer fresh berries like strawberries, blueberries, or raspberries with sugar-free yogurt or whipped cream in a glass or dish. This easy and delicious dessert is filled with antioxidants and fiber while being low in carbs.

7. Coconut Flour Pancakes: Coconut flour is a low-carb alternative to conventional flour and can be used to create excellent pancakes. Combine coconut flour with eggs, unsweetened almond milk, and a low-carb sweetener of your choosing. Top with sugar-free syrup or fresh berries.

8. Sugar-Free Popsicles: Make your own popsicles using sugar-free fruit juice or unsweetened tea. You may also add bits of fresh fruit or herbs like mint for extra taste. Homemade popsicles are a terrific way to cool off and enjoy a delicious treat without the extra sweets.

When cooking sugar-free and low-carb sweets, it is necessary to read labels carefully and pick sweeteners that are safe for those with diabetes.

Smart Snacking Tips for Blood Sugar Control

Managing blood sugar levels is critical for those with diabetes, and smart eating may play a big part in accomplishing this objective. By choosing the right snacks and following some essential tips, individuals can keep their blood sugar levels stable and prevent spikes or crashes. Here are some sensible eating suggestions for blood sugar management in a diabetic diet:

1. Opt for Low Glycemic Index (GI) Foods: The glycemic index evaluates how rapidly carbohydrates in diets elevate blood sugar levels. Choosing foods with a low glycemic index will help avoid unexpected rises in blood sugar. Examples of low

GI snacks include non-starchy veggies, nuts, seeds, and whole grains.

2. Combine carbs with Protein or Healthy Fats: Pairing carbs with protein or healthy fats will help slow down the absorption of glucose into the circulation, reducing abrupt spikes in blood sugar levels. For example, try an apple with a small handful of almonds or put some nut butter on whole grain crackers.

3. Watch Portion Sizes: Even healthy snacks might influence blood sugar levels if taken in big numbers. It is crucial to be cautious of portion proportions to prevent overeating and excessive carbohydrate consumption. Use measuring cups or a food scale to correctly measure out snacks and minimize mindless snacking.

4. Read Food Labels: When picking packaged snacks, it is vital to read food labels carefully. Look for snacks that are low in added sugars and rich in fiber. Avoid snacks that include high fructose corn syrup, artificial sweeteners, or bad fats like trans fats.

5. Plan Ahead: Planning snacks in advance might help folks make better choices and avoid reaching

for harmful alternatives when hunger hits. Prepare snack choices like pre-cut veggies, hard-boiled eggs, or portioned-out nuts and seeds to have on hand as required.

6. Stay Hydrated: Drinking adequate water throughout the day is vital for general health and may also help lower blood sugar levels. Sometimes, sensations of hunger might really be an indication of dehydration. Stay hydrated by drinking water or unsweetened liquids between snacks.

7. Listen to Your Body: Pay attention to your body's hunger and fullness signs. Snack when you are actually hungry, rather than out of boredom or habit. Practice mindful eating by eating deliberately and appreciating each mouthful, allowing your body to recognize when it is full.

8. Consult with a Healthcare Professional: Every individual's nutritional demands and objectives are unique. Consulting with a healthcare expert or registered dietitian may give tailored assistance on snack selections, portion management, and overall meal planning to help manage blood sugar levels.

Remember to pick snacks that are low in carbs, rich in fiber, protein, and healthy fats.

Meal Planning Tools and Resources

Grocery Shopping Tips for Diabetic Patients

Grocery shopping plays a critical part in treating diabetes and maintaining stable blood sugar levels. By making sensible decisions and following certain basic suggestions, persons with diabetes may ensure they enjoy a well-balanced and healthy diet. Here are some grocery shopping suggestions particularly targeted for diabetes patients:

1. write a List: Before traveling to the grocery shop, write a list of the products you need. This can help you remain focused and prevent impulsive purchases of unhealthy snacks or sugary meals. Include goods like fresh fruits and vegetables, lean meats, entire grains, and low-fat dairy products.

2. Shop the Perimeter: The perimeter of the grocery store is often where fresh vegetables, lean meats, and dairy goods are situated. Focus on browsing these regions since they tend to provide healthier selections compared to the central aisles that are full with processed and packaged items.

3. Choose Fresh Produce: Fill your cart with a choice of fresh fruits and veggies. These are low in calories, rich in fiber, and filled with important vitamins and minerals. Opt for bright alternatives like berries, leafy greens, bell peppers, and citrus fruits.

4. Look for Whole Grains: When choosing grains, consider whole grain alternatives such brown rice, quinoa, whole wheat bread, and whole grain pasta. These alternatives have more fiber and minerals compared to processed grains, which may help control blood sugar levels.

5. Read Food Labels: Reading food labels is vital when shopping for packaged goods. Look for goods that are low in added sugars, salt, and bad fats. Pay attention to the overall carbohydrate amount and pick those with greater fiber content.

6. Avoid Processed and Sugary Foods: Processed foods frequently include high quantities of added sugars, harmful fats, and salt. These may lead to blood sugar increases and severely damage general health. Opt for fresh, healthy foods whenever feasible.

7. Choose Lean Proteins: Include lean protein options in your grocery list, such as skinless fowl, fish, tofu, beans, and lentils. These selections are lower in saturated fats and might help keep you feeling full and pleased.

8. Stock Up on Healthy Fats: Include sources of healthy fats in your shopping basket, such as avocados, almonds, seeds, and olive oil. These fats may help enhance insulin sensitivity and boost heart health.

9. Be Mindful of Portion proportions: Pay attention to portion proportions when buying foods like nuts, nut butter, or dried fruits. These foods may be healthy options but should be taken in moderation owing to their calorie and carbohydrate levels.

10. Consider Frozen and Canned Options: Frozen fruits and vegetables may be a quick and healthy choice when fresh food is not easily accessible. Choose alternatives without added sweeteners or sauces. Canned meals like beans or tuna may also be healthy alternatives, but search for low-sodium varieties.

11. Don't Shop on an Empty Stomach: Shopping when hungry might lead to hasty purchasing of

unhealthy snacks or sugary meals. Eat a balanced supper or snack before going to the grocery shop to prevent making bad food choices.

12. Consult with a trained Dietitian: If you have unique dietary requirements or concerns, talking with a trained dietitian may give individualized counsel and assist build a meal plan that meets your individual needs and objectives.

By following these grocery shopping suggestions, persons with diabetes may make educated decisions that support their blood sugar management and general health. Remember to emphasize fresh, healthy foods, read food labels carefully, and speak with a healthcare expert for tailored recommendations.

Reading Food Labels for Diabetes-Friendly Choices

Reading food labels is a vital skill for those with diabetes who wish to make good decisions. When reading labels, it is vital to pay attention to the serving size, since this will impact the quantity of carbs and other nutrients eaten. The overall carbohydrate amount is particularly essential, since carbohydrates have the biggest influence on blood sugar levels. It is advisable to pick meals with a low glycemic index, which indicates they have a slower influence on blood sugar levels. Additionally, it is crucial to seek meals that are low in saturated and trans fats, since they might raise the risk of heart disease. Foods rich in fiber are especially useful for those with diabetes, since they may help manage blood sugar levels and promote digestion. Finally, it is crucial to avoid meals containing added sugars, since they may cause blood sugar levels to surge fast. By carefully reading food labels and selecting diabetic-friendly products, persons with diabetes may enjoy a nutritious and balanced diet.

Smart Grocery Shopping Strategies

Smart grocery shopping is vital for those with diabetes who wish to maintain a nutritious diet. When shopping for groceries, it is crucial to have a strategy and a list of nutritious things to purchase. This may help consumers avoid impulsive purchases and keep to their nutritional objectives. One approach for effective grocery shopping is to shop the perimeter of the store. This is where fresh vegetables, lean meats, and low-fat dairy items are often placed. Avoiding the middle aisles where processed and packaged goods are prevalent might help folks make better choices. When purchasing fruits and vegetables, it is crucial to choose a diversity of colors and varieties. This may guarantee that people obtain a diversity of vitamins, minerals, and antioxidants in their diet. It is also vital to pick whole grains, such as brown rice and quinoa, instead of refined grains like white bread and pasta.

Reading food labels is also vital for sensible supermarket shopping. As discussed before, patients with diabetes should pay attention to the portion size, total carbohydrate content, and glycemic index of meals. It is also crucial to seek foods that are low in saturated and trans fats, rich in fiber, and devoid of added sweets. It is necessary to plan ahead for meals and snacks. This may help folks avoid harmful decisions when they are hungry or short on time. Preparing meals in advance, carrying healthy snacks, and having a list of go-to dishes may all be beneficial tactics.

Wise grocery shopping methods for those with diabetes include browsing the perimeter of the store, picking a range of fruits and vegetables, selecting whole grains, reading product labels, and planning ahead for meals and snacks.

Meal Prep and Batch Cooking for Diabetic Patients

Benefits of Meal Prepping for Diabetes Management

Meal planning is a beneficial method for those with diabetes who wish to control their disease and keep a balanced diet. By preparing meals in advance, people may guarantee that they have nutritious alternatives accessible when they are hungry or short on time.

One advantage of meal prepping is that it may help folks regulate their portion sizes and prevent overeating. By measuring out portions ahead of time, people may guarantee that they are consuming the proper quantity of food to satisfy their nutritional objectives.

Meal preparation may also help consumers save money and prevent food waste. By purchasing materials in bulk and cooking meals in advance, folks may avoid consuming costly and harmful convenience foods. Additionally, meal preparation may help consumers use up items before they go bad, lowering the quantity of food that is wasted away.

Another advantage of meal preparing is that it might help consumers make better choices. By preparing meals in advance, people may ensure that they are eating a range of fruits, vegetables, lean meats, and healthy grains into their diet. This may help people satisfy their dietary requirements and lower their risk of developing issues associated with diabetes.

Meal preparation may help consumers save time and minimize stress. By preparing meals in advance, folks may avoid the stress of selecting what to eat at the last minute or hurrying to cook a meal after a hard day. This may help folks feel more comfortable and in control of their eating.

Meal prepping is a good method for those with diabetes who wish to control their disease and keep a nutritious diet. It may help consumers limit their portion sizes, save money and decrease food waste, make healthier choices, and save time and reduce stress.

Planning and Preparing Meals in Advance

Planning and preparing meals in advance is a beneficial method for those with diabetes who wish to control their condition and maintain a balanced diet. By taking the effort to plan out meals ahead of time, people may guarantee that they have nutritious alternatives accessible whether they are hungry or short on time.

One of the primary advantages of meal prepping is that it may help folks regulate their portion sizes and prevent overeating. This is particularly crucial for those with diabetes, since overeating may cause blood sugar levels to surge. By measuring out portions ahead of time, people may guarantee that they are consuming the proper quantity of food to satisfy their nutritional objectives.

Another advantage of meal prepping is that it may help consumers save money and prevent food waste. By purchasing materials in bulk and cooking meals in advance, folks may avoid consuming costly and harmful convenience foods. Additionally, meal preparation may help consumers use up items before they go bad, lowering the quantity of food that is wasted away.

Meal planning may also help consumers make better decisions. By preparing meals in advance, people may ensure that they are eating a range of fruits, vegetables, lean meats, and healthy grains into their diet. This may help people satisfy their dietary requirements and lower their risk of developing issues associated with diabetes.

Meal preparation may help consumers save time and minimize stress. By preparing meals in advance, folks may avoid the stress of selecting what to eat at the last minute or hurrying to cook a meal after a hard day. This may help folks feel more comfortable and in control of their eating.

Planning and preparing meals in advance is a good method for those with diabetes who wish to control their condition and maintain a nutritious diet. It may help consumers limit their portion sizes, save money and decrease food waste, make healthier choices, and save time and reduce stress.

Dining Out Guide for Diabetic Patients

Making Healthy Choices at Restaurants

Making smart choices at restaurants may be tough for persons with diabetes who wish to maintain a balanced diet. However, there are various ways that might help consumers make better choices while dining out. One of the first steps in choosing healthy selections at restaurants is to examine the menu ahead of time. Many restaurants now give nutrition information on their websites, which may help consumers make educated choices about what to purchase. By reading the menu in advance, consumers may select healthier alternatives and arrange their meal appropriately.

Another technique for choosing healthy selections at restaurants is to concentrate on lean meats, veggies, and whole grains. This may include selections such as grilled chicken or fish, salads with lean protein, and healthy grain side dishes. It is also crucial to avoid fried meals, creamy sauces, and high-calorie sweets, which might be heavy in fat and sugar. Portion management is especially vital while dining out. Many restaurants provide enormous quantities, which may contribute to overeating and rises in blood sugar levels. To prevent this, folks should ask for a lesser serving or share a meal with a friend or family member.

It is crucial to pay attention to beverages while dining out. Sugary drinks such as soda and juice may cause blood sugar levels to jump, thus it is recommended to stay with water or unsweetened beverages. Choosing healthy choices at restaurants may be tough for those with diabetes, but it is attainable with careful preparation and attention to menu alternatives. By concentrating on lean meats, vegetables, and whole grains, regulating portion sizes, and avoiding sugary beverages and high-calorie sweets, people may maintain a balanced diet when eating out. It is crucial to avoid fried dishes, creamy sauces, and high-calorie sweets, which might be heavy in fat and sugar. Portion management is particularly vital while dining out, since many restaurants provide huge amounts that may contribute to overeating and rises in blood sugar levels. To prevent this, folks should ask for a lesser serving or share a meal with a friend or family member.

Conclusion

Maintaining a Healthy Life, Regular Physical Activity and Diabetes Management

Regular physical exercise is an essential component of diabetes therapy. Exercise may help regulate blood sugar levels, enhance insulin sensitivity, and lower the risk of problems associated with diabetes. It is advised that patients with diabetes participate in at least 150 minutes of moderate-intensity aerobic activity each week, spaced out over at least three days. Aerobic activity, such as brisk walking, cycling, or swimming, may help reduce blood sugar levels by boosting the body's sensitivity to insulin. Resistance exercise, such as weightlifting, may also be advantageous by increasing muscle mass and enhancing glucose absorption. However, it is crucial to contact with a healthcare physician before beginning any fitness program, since some forms of exercise may not be good for those with particular health concerns.

In addition to increasing blood sugar management, regular physical exercise may also help manage other risk factors connected with diabetes, such as high blood pressure and high cholesterol. It may also enhance overall cardiovascular health and minimize the risk of heart disease. To include regular physical activity into their diabetes care plan, patients should start softly and progressively increase the intensity and duration of their exercise. They should also check their blood sugar levels before and after exercise to ensure they are within a healthy range. Additionally, it is crucial to keep hydrated and wear suitable footwear and clothes to avoid damage.

Generally, regular physical exercise is an essential part of diabetes care that may help patients maintain their blood sugar levels and enhance their general health.

Stress Management and Sleep Importance

Stress and lack of sleep may have a severe influence on blood sugar levels and general health for those with diabetes. Therefore, stress management and obtaining appropriate sleep are crucial components of diabetes control. Stress may cause the body to produce hormones that raise blood sugar levels. This may be particularly troublesome for those with diabetes who already have problems managing their blood sugar levels. Stress management practices such as deep breathing, meditation, and exercise may help lower stress levels and improve blood sugar control. In addition to stress management, obtaining adequate sleep is also vital for those with diabetes. Lack of sleep may induce insulin resistance, making it more difficult for the body to control blood sugar levels. It may also lead to increased hunger and desires for unhealthy foods, which can further adversely influence blood sugar regulation.

To enhance sleep quality, persons with diabetes should attempt to maintain a regular sleep pattern and adopt a pleasant nighttime ritual. They should also avoid coffee and alcohol before night, since these might impair sleep. Additionally, it is necessary to ensure that the resting environment is pleasant and favorable to sleep. Stress management and obtaining appropriate sleep are crucial parts of diabetes care that may help patients control their blood sugar levels and improve their overall health. By implementing these behaviors into their daily routine, persons with diabetes may enhance their quality of life and lower the risk of complications connected with the illness.

Ongoing Monitoring and Support

Ongoing monitoring and support are crucial for persons with diabetes to manage their illness properly. Regular monitoring of blood sugar levels, blood pressure, cholesterol levels, and weight may assist patients with diabetes discover any changes or trends that may necessitate revisions to their treatment plan. Support from family and friends may also be useful for those with diabetes. Loved ones may give support and incentive to keep to a healthy lifestyle and treatment plan. They may also assist persons with diabetes manage stress and deal with the difficulties of living with a chronic disease.

Technology may also play a role in continual monitoring and assistance for patients with diabetes. Continuous glucose monitoring devices and insulin pumps may give real-time data on blood sugar levels and insulin administration, enabling patients make educated choices regarding their treatment. Constant monitoring and assistance are necessary for persons with diabetes to manage their illness successfully and limit the risk of complications. By working closely with healthcare providers, loved ones, and leveraging technology, persons with diabetes may take charge of their health and enhance their quality of life.

Sample Meal Plans for Different Caloric Needs

1200-Calorie Diabetic Meal Plan

Sample meal ideas for a 1200-calorie diabetic meal plan:

Day 1: - Breakfast: 1 small whole wheat English muffin, 1 scrambled egg, 1 slice of low-fat cheese, ½ cup of blueberries
- Snack: 1 tiny apple, 1 spoonful of almond butter
- Lunch: 2 cups of mixed greens, ½ cup of cherry tomatoes, 3 ounces of grilled chicken breast, 2 teaspoons of balsamic vinaigrette dressing
- Snack: 1 tiny orange, 10 unsalted almonds
- Dinner: 3 ounces of grilled salmon, 1 cup of steamed broccoli, ½ cup of cooked brown rice

Day 2: - Breakfast: 1 small whole wheat bagel, 1 spoonful of cream cheese, 1 tiny banana
- Snack: 1 small pear, 1 low-fat string cheese -
Lunch: 2 cups of vegetable soup, 3 whole grain crackers, 1 small apple
- Snack: 1 tiny peach, 10 unsalted pistachios
- Dinner: 3 ounces of grilled chicken breast, 1 cup of roasted Brussels sprouts, ½ cup of cooked quinoa

Day 3: - Breakfast: 1 small whole wheat tortilla, 1 scrambled egg, ¼ avocado, salsa, 1 tiny orange
- Snack: 1 tiny apple, 1 spoonful of peanut butter
- Lunch: 2 cups of mixed greens, ½ cup of cherry tomatoes, 3 ounces of grilled shrimp, 2 teaspoons of lemon vinaigrette dressing
- Snack: 1 tiny banana, 10 unsalted cashews
- Dinner: 3 ounces of grilled sirloin steak, 1 cup of roasted asparagus, ½ cup of boiled sweet potato

1500-Calorie Diabetic Meal Plan

Sample meal ideas for a 1500-calorie diabetic meal plan:

Day 1: - Breakfast: 1 small whole wheat English muffin, 1 scrambled egg, 1 slice of low-fat cheese, ½ cup of blueberries, 1 cup of unsweetened almond milk
- Snack: 1 tiny apple, 1 spoonful of almond butter
- Lunch: 2 cups of mixed greens, ½ cup of cherry tomatoes, 3 ounces of grilled chicken breast, 2 teaspoons of balsamic vinaigrette sauce, 1 small whole wheat roll - Snack: 1 small orange, 10 unsalted almonds
- Dinner: 3 ounces of grilled salmon, 1 cup of steamed broccoli, ½ cup of cooked brown rice, 1 small whole wheat dinner roll

Day 2: - Breakfast: 1 small whole wheat bagel, 1 spoonful of cream cheese, 1 small banana, 1 cup of unsweetened almond milk
- Snack: 1 small pear, 1 low-fat string cheese - Lunch: 2 cups of vegetable soup, 3 whole grain crackers, 1 small apple, 1 small whole wheat roll - Snack: 1 small peach, 10 unsalted pistachios
- Dinner: 3 ounces of grilled chicken breast, 1 cup of roasted Brussels sprouts, ½ cup of boiled quinoa, 1 small whole wheat dinner roll

Day 3: - Breakfast: 1 small whole wheat tortilla, 1 scrambled egg, ¼ avocado, salsa, 1 tiny orange, 1 cup of unsweetened almond milk
- Snack: 1 tiny apple, 1 spoonful of peanut butter
- Lunch: 2 cups of mixed greens, ½ cup of cherry tomatoes, 3 ounces of grilled shrimp, 2 teaspoons of lemon vinaigrette dressing, 1 small whole wheat roll
- Snack: 1 small banana, 10 unsalted cashews
- Dinner: 3 ounces of grilled sirloin steak, 1 cup of roasted asparagus, ½ cup of boiled sweet potato, 1 small whole wheat dinner roll

1800-Calorie Diabetic Meal Plan

Day 1:
- Breakfast: 1 small whole wheat English muffin, 1 scrambled egg, 1 slice of low-fat cheese, ½ cup of blueberries, 1 cup of unsweetened almond milk

- Snack: 1 small apple, 1 spoonful of nut butter -
Lunch: 2 cups of mixed greens, ½ cup of cherry
tomatoes, 3 ounces of grilled chicken breast, 2
teaspoons of balsamic vinaigrette dressing, 1 small
whole wheat roll - Snack: 1 small orange, 10
unsalted almonds
- Dinner: 3 ounces of grilled salmon, 1 cup of
steamed broccoli, ½ cup of cooked brown rice, 1
small whole wheat dinner roll

Day 2: - Breakfast: 1 small whole wheat bagel, 1
spoonful of cream cheese, 1 small banana, 1 cup of
unsweetened almond milk
- Snack: 1 small pear, 1 low-fat string cheese -
Lunch: 2 cups of vegetable soup, 3 whole grain
crackers, 1 small apple, 1 small whole wheat roll -
Snack: 1 small peach, 10 unsalted pistachios
- Dinner: 3 ounces of grilled chicken breast, 1 cup of
roasted Brussels sprouts, ½ cup of boiled quinoa, 1
small whole wheat dinner roll

Day 3: - Breakfast: 1 small whole wheat tortilla, 1
scrambled egg, ¼ avocado, salsa, 1 tiny orange, 1
cup of unsweetened almond milk
- Snack: 1 tiny apple, 1 spoonful of peanut butter
- Lunch: 2 cups of mixed greens, ½ cup of cherry
tomatoes, 3 ounces of grilled shrimp, 2 teaspoons of

lemon vinaigrette dressing, 1 small whole wheat roll
- Snack: 1 small banana, 10 unsalted cashews
- Dinner: 3 ounces of grilled sirloin steak, 1 cup of roasted asparagus, ½ cup of boiled sweet potato, 1 small whole wheat dinner roll

2000-Calorie Diabetic Meal Plan

Day 1:
- Breakfast: 1 small whole wheat English muffin, 1 scrambled egg, 1 slice of low-fat cheese, ½ cup of blueberries, 1 cup of unsweetened almond milk
- Snack: 1 small apple, 1 spoonful of nut butter - Lunch: 2 cups of mixed greens, ½ cup of cherry tomatoes, 3 ounces of grilled chicken breast, 2 teaspoons of balsamic vinaigrette dressing, 1 small whole wheat roll - Snack: 1 small orange, 10 unsalted almonds
- Dinner: 3 ounces of grilled salmon, 1 cup of steamed broccoli, ½ cup of cooked brown rice, 1 small whole wheat dinner roll

Day 2: - Breakfast: 1 small whole wheat bagel, 1 spoonful of cream cheese, 1 small banana, 1 cup of unsweetened almond milk
- Snack: 1 small pear, 1 low-fat string cheese - Lunch: 2 cups of vegetable soup, 3 whole grain crackers, 1 small apple, 1 small whole wheat roll - Snack: 1 small peach, 10 unsalted pistachios

- Dinner: 3 ounces of grilled chicken breast, 1 cup of roasted Brussels sprouts, ½ cup of boiled quinoa, 1 small whole wheat dinner roll

Day 3: - Breakfast: 1 small whole wheat tortilla, 1 scrambled egg, ¼ avocado, salsa, 1 tiny orange, 1 cup of unsweetened almond milk
- Snack: 1 tiny apple, 1 spoonful of peanut butter
- Lunch: 2 cups of mixed greens, ½ cup of cherry tomatoes, 3 ounces of grilled shrimp, 2 teaspoons of lemon vinaigrette dressing, 1 small whole wheat roll
- Snack: 1 small banana, 10 unsalted cashews
- Dinner: 3 ounces of grilled sirloin steak, 1 cup of roasted asparagus, ½ cup of boiled sweet potato, 1 small whole wheat dinner roll

It is crucial to remember that these meal plans are simply suggestions and may need to be altered depending on individual requirements and tastes. It is also crucial to contact a healthcare expert, such as a qualified dietitian, before making any substantial modifications to your diet.

Frequently Asked Questions about Diabetes and Meal Planning

1. What is diabetes?

Diabetes is a chronic illness that affects the way the body handles blood sugar (glucose). There are two forms of diabetes: Type 1 and Type 2.

2. What is blood sugar management?

Blood sugar management includes maintaining blood sugar levels within a healthy range by food, exercise, and medication.

3. What are carbohydrates?

Carbohydrates are one of the three macronutrients (together with protein and fat) that supply energy to the body. They are found in meals including bread, pasta, grains, fruits, and vegetables.

4. What is the glycemic index?

The glycemic index is a rating system that analyzes how rapidly carbohydrates in meals elevate blood sugar levels. those with a high glycemic index (such as white bread and sugary beverages) cause blood sugar to jump fast, whereas those with a low glycemic index (such as whole grains and vegetables) produce a longer, more steady increase in blood sugar.

5. What function do fiber, protein, and fat play in blood sugar control?

Fiber, protein, and fat all slow down the absorption of carbs in the body, which helps to manage blood sugar levels. Foods strong in fiber (such as whole grains and vegetables), protein (such as lean meats and legumes), and healthy fats (such as nuts and avocado) are crucial components of a balanced diet for diabetic treatment.

6. How may portion control and serving sizes assist with diabetes management?

Eating too much food at once might cause blood sugar levels to surge. Portion management and following suggested serving sizes may assist to keep blood sugar levels constant.

7. What is glycemic load?

Glycemic load takes into consideration both the glycemic index of a meal and the serving size. It gives a more precise indication of how a specific meal may effect blood sugar levels.

8. What are some ideas for meal planning for diabetes?

Some ideas for meal planning for diabetes include: selecting foods with a low glycemic index, integrating fiber, protein, and healthy fats in meals, controlling portion sizes, and preparing meals in advance.

9. What are some breakfast dishes for regulated blood sugar levels?

Some breakfast dishes for regulated blood sugar levels include: oatmeal with nuts and berries, Greek yogurt with fruit and granola, and scrambled eggs with veggies.

10. What are good lunch dishes for regulated blood sugar levels?

Some lunch ideas for balanced blood sugar levels include: turkey and avocado wrap, quinoa salad with veggies and poultry, and lentil soup with whole grain bread.

11. What are some supper dishes for regulated blood sugar levels?

Some supper dishes for regulated blood sugar levels include: grilled salmon with roasted vegetables, baked chicken with sweet potato and green beans, and stir-fry with tofu and vegetables.

12. What are good snacks and sweets for balanced blood sugar levels?

Some snacks and sweets for regulated blood sugar levels include: apple slices with almond butter, Greek yogurt with berries, and dark chocolate with almonds.

13. How can persons with diabetes handle special events like vacations and parties?

People with diabetes may handle special events by planning ahead, limiting portion sizes, selecting meals with a low glycemic index, and keeping physically active.

14. What are some suggestions for eating out with diabetes?

Some advice for eating out with diabetes include: reviewing restaurant menus in advance, asking for substitutes or alterations to meals, and controlling portion sizes.

15. How may exercise and physical activity assist with blood sugar control?

Exercise and physical exercise may assist to reduce blood sugar levels by increasing insulin sensitivity and enhancing glucose absorption by the muscles. Regular exercise may also assist to maintain a healthy weight and lower the risk of problems from diabetes.